AF651873

DESIGNING HRD SYSTEMS

By the same Author:

1. Dynamics of Formulating Policy in Government of India: Machinery for Policy Development (Concept, 1976)
2. Change in Work Organisation: Some Experience of Renewal in Social Systems (Concept, 1977)
3. Organization for Management in Developing Countries (Concept, 1983)
4. Organising Innovation: A Management Study (Concept, 1991)

About the Author

The Author is Professor Emeritus at the Management Development Institute, Gurgaon. He completed his assignment as Founder Director of the fourth national level Institute of Management at Lucknow in July 1988. Prior to this; Chief Technical Adviser, International Labour Organization in Lagos, Nigeria; Director, Indian Institute of Public Administration, New Delhi and Senior Professor at Indian Institute of Management at Calcutta and later in Ahmedabad. Prof. Dayal came to teaching in 1963 after having worked for about 15 years in senior managerial positions in industry.

Prof. Dayal has been consultant to many large organizations in India such as Life Insurance Corporation, Air India, Indian Airlines, Mafatlal Industries, Balmer Lawrie Group, DCM and others. He has served on several commissions and committees of the Union and State Governments.

Prof. Dayal has served on the Corporate Boards of several organizations such as Bharat Electronics Ltd., Indo-Burmah Petroleum, Indian Oil Corporation, National Textile Corporation and others.

Prof. Dayal has published 22 books and monographs and over 250 papers in journals and periodicals in India and abroad.

DESIGNING HRD SYSTEMS

ISHWAR DAYAL
Professor Emeritus
Management Development Institute
Gurgaon

CONCEPT PUBLISHING COMPANY PVT. LTD.
NEW DELHI-110059

© Ishwar Dayal (*b*. 1924-)

All rights reserved. No part of this work may be reproduced, stored, adapted, or transmitted in any form or by any means, electronic, mechanical, photocopying, micro-filming recording or otherwise, or translated in any language, without the prior written permission of the copyright owner and the publisher. The book is sold subject to the condition that it shall not, by way of trade or otherwise, be lent, resold, hired out, or otherwise circulated without the prior publisher's written consent in any form of binding or cover other than that in which it is published.

The views and opinions expressed in this book are editor(s) own and the facts reported by him/her have been verified to the extent possible, and the publishers are not in any way liable for the same.

ISBN: 978-81-7022-456-3

First Published 1993

Published and Printed by

Concept
Since 1974

Concept Publishing Company Pvt. Ltd.
A/15-16, Commercial Block, Mohan Garden,
New Delhi-110059 (India)
T : 91-11-41101460
E : publishing@conceptpub.com, *W*: www.conceptpub.com

CONTENTS

PREFACE

One chief executive recently remarked that he found it difficult to imagine how people in his position managed their business earlier without extensive consultative arrangements that they incorporated two years ago. The understanding between the management and the employees has grown during this period and the company has been able to rationalize their operating systems to bring out a better product, reduce the cost of production and offer higher quality of customer service.

A large number of studies of management of successful corporations in India and abroad also show that involvement of employees in work is essential for improving performance. But the way to achieve this is by no means clear. And this has indeed been the core concern of a great deal of management action from early Western Electric experiments in the twenties to the present day. Gandhiji promoted the idea of trusteeship. He believed that the management should consider themselves as trustees of society for whose benefit the enterprise was created. According to this concept the management and the employees have the same goal, and they share responsibility for the well-being of society. To achieve this goal, cooperation between all sections of employees is essential. But this concept is generally not accepted intellectually by the management or the union, nor is it practised.

Human Resource Development (HRD) approaches broadly seek involvement of employees at work and they are linked to growth and development of individuals. It is assumed that most people will take greater responsibility for results when they have autonomy, self-reliance and confidence at work. While the nature of HRD interventions differ from one organization to another, they have, generally, growth orientation common to most.

This book includes seven papers on different aspects of HRD interventions. Five of these papers were published earlier. Three papers have been revised extensively and the other two are edited to make them suitable for the present volume. Two other papers are written exclusively for this book. I am grateful to the publishers of the earlier papers for giving me permission to use them in this volume. These sources are acknowledged in each case.

I thank K.V.L.N. Murthy and N.J. Singh for their help in typing the manuscript.

NEW DELHI
December 1992

ISHWAR DAYAL

1

PLANNING HRD INITIATIVES*

One of the most respected scholars in management, Fritz Roethlisberger of Harvard University, had visualized the task of management as generating spontaneous will to cooperate. From early 40s when Roethlisberger first wrote about this, many approaches have been devised to achieve this purpose. The search for ways that would serve this purpose have continued. Human Resource Development (HRD) is yet another approach to develop a healthy and purposeful human organization in an enterprise.

The studies of successful organizations over the past 15-20 years also highlight the fact that improved performance has always accompanied the involvement of people at work. No improvement in organizational performance is possible without such involvement. The Japanese experience has reconfirmed the need for such engagement.

I believe that the experience of industrialized countries in this respect is equally valid for India and our efforts to improve organizational performance will depend largely on how effective the management is in generating spontaneous will to cooperate among employees. In this chapter I have assumed that this proposition is valid. I have, therefore, examined the considerations that would help organizations build a healthy human system. Any

---

* Revised. Original prepared for keynote address at the Annual Conference of Insurance Institute of India held in New Delhi on September 27, 1992.

planning exercise has to take into account the basic data about whatever we are planning, and the strategy that would help us reach the goal we may wish to reach.

The basic premise for HRD is man's knowledge of himself — his nature and how and why he responds to his situation and the people with whom he interacts. These data must be taken into consideration in formulating a plan of action in an organization. The theme of this chapter is how these data should be applied to planning HRD system in an organization.

Human beings have certain unique characteristics. Some of them are:

(i) Capability for improving his own understanding and performance.
(ii) Versatility that no other animate being or inanimate object has.
(iii) Ability to be a prime-mover in whatever capacity he is involved.
(iv) Capability to go beyond set structures of thinking and doing, of being innovative and covering new ground.
(v) Ability to change himself if he were to feel the need for doing so.

Notwithstanding these qualities, a human being could function like a machine with a highly structured area of thinking and doing. His mechanical orientation could induce rigidity in his approach and performance. With age mental alertness and physical energy may deteriorate but until a fairly advanced age, maturity and the capacity to objectively evaluate events remains sharp and, in many cases, improves.

This is the circumstance relating to people. The term resource in relation to people, indicates that they are a resource in themselves, which they can either appreciate or depreciate, depending upon what they do with themselves. In common use human resources is a term used to refer to the numbers of employees at work. In this meaning, a person is seen much the same way as physical assets such as a table or a machine. In another meaning, however, human resource is used to refer to the quality of the person, and his contribution to organizational effectiveness. The second meaning applies to HRD initiatives.

Another difference between physical and human assets is significant and need mention. The physical and financial assets respond to direct action by the manager; this is not the case with human assets. Managerial action is interpreted through the sentiments and feelings that constitute the intervening variable in his response. This difference between physical and human assets is becoming clearer over the years through research and systematic study of experience at work. This difference, in fact, constitutes the foundation for human relations approach in organizations. People can become an asset, a liability or a block depending on how they themselves, as individuals and groups, experience the situation where they are placed.

Another human characteristic is that an individual reacts to people and situations. It is not a stationary state. A person does well in an organization *A* and the same person does poorly in a similar situation in organization *B*. He gets along well with one supervisor or a colleague but not with another supervisor and another colleague. He interprets one statement from one manager favourably but suspects the same statement from another manager. It is not the statement *per se* but the totality of the situation that guides the interpretation of what is said and what is heard. Roethlisberger (1942, p. 10) refers to this as follows:

> "The feeling and sentiments people have and the values and assumptions they hold tend to affect the way they see things about them" and later, "I realize I should not belabour this commonplace observation. All of us have had enough experience to realise that we do not perceive the reality quite the same way as our parents, our teachers, our bosses, our wives, or our children. And yet it is curious how in the heat of controversy we forget this fact when it is more important for us to remember it."

It is also observed that this fact is often overlooked in formulating personnel or human relations policies or approaches and practices. Analysis of personnel policies in five organizations regarded as leaders show that assumptions underlying the policies generally ignored the data obtained in behaviour studies, or in common experience. Rather, the assumption made in these organizations is that everyone has the same needs and everyone should fit into the set of rules formulated to regulate behaviour. The experience also shows that the more rigid the rules, the more formal and "legalistic" is the relationship (Dayal, 1967). An organization such as CMC, recognizing differential responses and differential patterns of human needs, has instituted personnel practices that are different from those found in the organizations mentioned above. All privileges apply to all categories to employees. If someone has an urgent need he is free to go out and come back. There is no laid down rule defining casual leave eligibility. A person can take leave according to his requirements. Interestingly enough the total number of days of leave taken per employee in CMC is lower than the days taken in most organizations. Similar considerations have given rise to many innovative practices abroad such as responsibility for results being pushed down the hierarchy, control through results

(Tannenbaum, 1962; McGregor, 1966; Whyte, 1959) flexi time system, greater autonomy at work, etc.

Briefly many organizations have begun to recognize the behavioural characteristics and the implications of these in policy formulation. One manifestation of this development is what has come to be generally known as Human Resource Development.

Knowledge about human behaviour is obtained from many sources. Bennis writes (1967, p. 10):

- From psychology we have psychoanalytic, role and cognitive theories;
- From sociology there are bureaucratic, social-system, symbolic interactionism and role theories;
- From anthropology have sprung the central ideas of norms, sentiments cohesion and interaction;
- From political science has come the recent work on conflict theory;
- From economics the decision processes and choice mechanism have been elucidated;
- From the historical approach have come mainly case studies which have helped to clarify the role of key decision-makers."

Integration of knowledge from many social sciences and research has helped our understanding of what has been referred to in literature as a complex man.

The complex nature of man suggests that behaviour is not guided by a simple stimulus-response relationship. A person may respond differently to the same stimulus in two different situations, or at different times. There is an intervening variable which would change the response. The intervening variable is the sentiment or the feelings of the respondent in a given situation. The sentiments and behaviour has to be studied in totality, and not as isolated events or factors. This is one aspect of relationship that accounts for the complexity of man. Having stated this, the research data also suggest that behavioural response is consistent; it has a pattern. A person under similar conditions responds in the same way. And a careful study of these patterns could help in predicting behaviour. This is the essence of understanding behaviour in organizations.

Now the question is what has this concept to do with management, or managing people in organizations. The discussion on behaviour so far suggests that the source of energy which motivates an individual to act lies within himself. He forms opinions or his views of the organizational life by interacting with his peers, superiors and people who are seen to have power in that system. The discussion here provides a generalized picture about human behaviour. It states only the basic formulation about how people behave. There are individual differences depending upon a specific background of community, family and unique experience in one's life, or in the process of growing up. These areas constitute the study of human personality. Before we examine the implication of behavioural data we need to raise another question. If behaviour is inner oriented, how do individuals learn new ways or bring about change in their behaviour in organizations. Broadly a person would strive to change his behaviour if he were to feel or perceive the need to do so. The need could arise due to his own experience, or influence of people he holds in high esteem, or persuasion of a referrent group, or a combination of several other factors. Even when the need is felt or perceived, the individual's involvement grows out of doing things himself, and by achieving success in new behaviour. His experience leads to a conviction and a belief. A change in the way of doing things at work, for example, would require that the person first sees that there is need to do work in a different way and that there may be a better way of doing it. He should perceive some merit in following a different way. By achieving a certain measure of success in following the new way he develops a feeling that the new way serves better than the old. This perception leads to his conviction about the new way of work. These are the processes through which a person changes his work habit, and adopts new styles. A strategy for initiating whatever change the organization desires will have to include these considerations. How best an organization will deal with each or all these aspects will depend upon the history, culture and environment of the organization concerned.

Most other resources can be developed by direct intervention of the management. Inventory can be increased or decreased, or money can be borrowed or generated by some action that management might take, but in developing human resources action has to be in terms of generating a process by which the individual concerned can enhance his own perspective or capability. The nature of intervention in HRD is *process intervention* and, therefore, we need to explore what aspects of management work generate the appropriate process for human growth. The action is indirect as compared to action that enhances other resources in the enterprise.

Having examined the salient features of human behaviour, we have to raise three different kinds, but related questions:

(i) What bearing has this discussion on HRD?
(ii) What should be the focus of an HRD initiative?
(iii) What is the link between HRD and personnel functions?

(i) Bearing on HRD

What is HRD? As development of human resource is different from material, financial or any other kind of resource, appreciation of the human resource means that a person becomes more capable of handling his affairs, or basically improves his capability for decision-making. He gains confidence in his capabilities. In some cases his personal skill needed for his job becomes sharper. Unlike other resources, however, the effort for appreciating the capability is basically that of the individual. This power is activated in certain environment and decelerates in certain other environment. A primary function of an HRD exercise in an organization is to undertake those aspects of work life which would create the environment or initiate managerial practices that would facilitate this process, and encourage it. Briefly HRD implies that the organization wants to enhance the overall capabilities of its employees to develop their potential in directions best suited to them.

Question is often asked why an organization should take up an exercise that sounds like one leading primary to self-development. Two aspects need to be considered:

(i) Organizations have found that the trickle-down effect of self-growth is many-sided and not least of this is on an individual's behaviour. Growth constitutes the intervening variable in stimulus-response relationship; the sentiment generally spreads over to his performance of the organizational tasks, and

(ii) The activities undertaken for self-improvement invariably focus around the specific problem areas of the organization. These problems invariably involve people and many of these problems find solution as a part of the HRD exercise. Efforts have been made to automate or robotize operating systems. All such measures have changed the requirements of skills of those who are engaged on operating jobs, and the skills of supervisory people, but it would appear that human element will always be critical in operations. In service industry the human factor has become more important than ever before.

Expectations of people are constantly changing and wherever their involvement in work is considered necessary, the management will have to evolve ways of responding to these needs in constructive and comprehensive ways. In realistic terms human involvement or generating a spontaneous will to cooperate has to be a central concern of enterprise management. Viewed from this perspective, the question is what has the management to do to obtain the involvement of employees, rather than why need it be concerned about doing so.

Once this proposition is accepted, the problem of individual growth becomes important, because involvement without growth is unlikely. The orientation of the individual, uniqueness and need satisfaction are the means through which involvement at work are likely to result. Thus a strategy for Human Resource Development in an organization may have to use these as a foundation.

(ii) Focus of an HRD Programme

In many organizations managers invariably claim that they are doing so much for employees but their performance shows little improvement. I think we are used to thinking in terms of mechanistic and simple as against complex formulations about social events. Mechanistic approach would imply that applying *n* units of pressure should shift an object to *y* distance, and *2n* units should shift it to *2y* distance. A simple formulation about an event suggests that in response to my giving *p* units, the individual should derive *q* units of sentiments. *2p* units should yield *2q* units. Intellectually most of us recognize that such mechanistic formulations are not valid or even realistic. Yet in policy formulation in many organizations this knowledge or awareness is seldom reflected. One highly successful chief executive wanted us to examine why employees hold negative feelings about the organization even when the management had done so much about their welfare. They had given extra benefits, such as housing, retirement benefits, holidays and other amenities which compared favourably with other comparable organizations. We often ignore that these measures cannot be motivational, except when need for them is felt at a given point of time. A satisfied need is not a motivator. Hence motivational strategies that rely on physical or extrinsic factors are unlikely to serve long-term involvement of employees (McGregor, 1960). Hence HRD has to look for intrinsic factors where the individual himself is a party to his own development, and these will have to rely primarily on what Herzberg (1966) has called motivating factors.

What should then be the focus of an HRD programme? The discussion so far suggests that the focus would have to be the growth of the individual. The term growth is used here to include adjustment to one's situation, capability to handle his affairs, wider awareness of the environment, skills and enhanced personal capabilities. An interesting example comes from an organization in Bombay. The company had a history of poor labour-management relations. The management started training programmes for workers in small batches. They put down a condition that the training programme will not have anything to do with his work; it will cover some information about the company but more specifically, material for his general knowledge, how to prepare family budget, child-rearing practices, etc Towards the end of the programme, families of workers were encouraged to come specially to learn about child-rearing practices, family budgets, etc. The organization arranged many programmes of this nature. After a few groups had gone through the programme, other employees asked when they would be nominated for training. Among other things, the labour-management relations in this organization improved dramatically and the productivity went up way beyond their expectations. The concept of growth for this organization is growth of a person as a total being and not only improvement in his skills or work-related behaviour. HRD has to be concerned with the individual as a person, and not "a split person as an employee alone". The implication of this approach is that even if one is organizing a training programme, it should include aspects that relate to personal growth. The training, by and large, should have development orientation and not that of skill alone. This concern would have to spread to problem-solving, decision-making, supervisory practices, and all other aspects of business. It should become a philosophy of work and not a technique.

(iii) The Link between HRD and Personnel

The link is important for the organization. Many years ago, McGregor (1961, 1966) had shown that underlying a policy decision is an assumption about people. A policy decision leads to a set of procedures and practices, which in turn influence how people react to the procedure or the practice. Resensweig refers to it as a self-fulfilling prophecy. One assumes that an employee needs close supervision and sets up practices to do so. When the employee shows signs of shirking work, one reiterates the decision for close supervision, though shirking work may be a reaction to close supervision, and not to his *basic* human nature.

In established organizations, practices and procedures grow and qualifications to rules are almost constantly added. This process assumes almost alarming proportions in large bureaucratic organizations, though the phenomenon is universal. Whatever rationale may have governed the initial formulation of personnel rules and regulations, over the years, that rationale is often compromised or becomes diffused. HRD approaches suggest that personnel practices are carefully studied to examine how consistent with the philosophy are the assumptions underlying the policy or the practices. The practices are meant to facilitate behaviour but often they become an end in themselves.

Strictly HRD is not a function but an approach. It is meaningful when it is applied by all managers right across the organization. It is a belief that under certain circumstances people are capable of improving their capability. This belief has to be reflected in dealing with people, supervision and, as mentioned earlier, in problem-solving and decision-making. The implementation of HRD programmes would have to be carried out by managers, though policy and strategy would need a specialist to do the job. In some organizations the specialist is attached to the Personnel Department provided the Head of Personnel holds a senior management position. In organizations where personnel function has low developmental and high fire-fighting orientation, the HRD specialist invariably reports direct to the Chief Executive. The job of the specialist will include helping the top management formulate an HRD policy, evolve an appropriate strategy, education of managers at all levels, implementation of the ideas and programmes at all levels, and review of effectiveness of the policy. Personally I favour HRD specialist being a part of the

Personnel Department where this function is given near top level status and has the perspective of development as against that of routinization of establishment matters. These decisions would vary from one organization to another and from one period of time to another.

The premises outlined above help us to generalize the features of HRD in an organization, whatever the nature of the programme.

1. HRD is founded on the belief that people are capable of growth and that management has to create an environment of growth. In many cases the growth experience will lead to an employee's involvement at work. This belief has to be manifested in managerial practices and in the behaviour of managers and supervisors who are the key agents of HRD in the organization. The belief about people has to be widely shared by key functionaries and not by a scattered few in the organization.

2. For operational purposes, large organizations use anchor points for developing HRD thrust. These areas are those that provide a direct link with development of individuals. Generally these areas concern career planning, appraisal, training, counselling, communication practices, supervision and growth orientation in problem-solving and decision-making. The choice of anchor points is determined on the basis of immediacy of problems that the organization experiences. These vary substantially from one organization to another.

3. The involvement of an individual in his own growth is an essential condition of growth. The individual has to recognize areas of improvement, carry out such activities as would develop these aspects and review how well his efforts are successful in serving the intended purpose. This is generally the cycle that facilitates growth. In a number of organizations jobs have to be re-designed to allow this kind of planning and review to take place. In this respect organizational development efforts in an

organization link well with HRD initiatives.

HRD programmes vastly vary in nature. Some include all the features that are identified here and some others include one or another aspect. There are some others which equate training with HRD. In a large number of HRD initiatives, the rationale or the underlying assumptions are vague or unspecific. Programmes undertaken without clarity of goal become a series of activities which may or may not lead to organizational effectiveness.

Some Approaches

The approaches to HRD are governed by the particular orientation of the management, its history and the kind of problems that it faces. In our studies we have found that the programmes vary significantly in their approach, and emphasis.* Broadly the emphasis may be classified in three respects as follows:

(i) Emphasis on Philosophy
(ii) Emphasis on Programmes
(iii) Emphasis on Leader Behaviour

(i) *Emphasis on Philosophy*

Some organizations have articulated their beliefs about people and have operationalized them in personnel systems and managerial practices in the organization. Two clear examples of these in our sample are CMC and Eicher. Their practices are people-oriented. The logic of

---

* This section is based mainly on data from the Project on HRD at the Management Development Institute, Gurgaon, undertaken by a team consisting of Ishwar Dayal, Punam Sahgal, Parvinder Kaur, A.K. Sen and Rashmi Jain. The findings are briefly reported in an article by Sahgal and Jain (1992).

their approach will broadly be thus: If we have faith in our employees, how should we treat them? We should share our ideas with them, respect their opinions and sensibilities, give them freedom to decide upon things that concern them, allow them to be responsible for results and so on. Our relationships and our managerial practices should be governed by these considerations. The personnel practices should assume that they are adults and would normally behave in ways that are in the best interest of the corporation. It is possible that some individuals would deviate from what is expected of them but for the sake of a few exceptions, the majority should not be put in a strait-jacket. These stray cases should be handled as cases and in best possible ways. Such organizations generally do not make a distinction between what is commonly found in India, Class I, II, III and IV. Organizations such as CMC and Eicher have to review their beliefs and examine the implications of these beliefs on a regular basis. CMC, for example, do it in their top and senior management seminars, keep their doors open for people to say what they feel and take corrective measures wherever necessary. Eicher do it through carefully planned employee surveys and use the data to evaluate how well the system is operating.

HRD is not seen to be a programme but a way of life. The sentiment pervades through the entire organization and covers all employees. HRD in such organizations is measured in terms of how seriously employees involve themselves in the affairs of the corporation, and how they show responsibility for the tasks they perform. Employees do not wait for instructions from higher levels – they take decisions and consult superiors where they feel help is needed. Emphasis in this approach is on the appropriateness of the managerial systems.

(ii) *Emphasis on Programmes*

Most organizations integrate their HRD initiatives with the problem areas identified by them. ITC had need for managers with diverse capabilities for their diversification programme. The initial thrust in their HRD initiatives was appraisal training and decentralization of responsibility for results. The programme spread later to all areas of significance. Crompton Greaves had need for geographical dispersal and emphasized role clarity and autonomy at managerial levels.

E.I.D. Parry likewise had to rehabilitate the company from a state of sickness and felt that building up the employee morale and trust in management were necessary. They initiated several policy measures and started intensive training programmes from higher to lower levels of management. Their effort was to create a family-like relationship which included concern for helping families to solve their problems such as family budgets, alcoholism and the like. The management clearly articulated the goal, but the programmes to achieve the purpose developed as the need was felt and the problems got identified. In all these efforts three aspects are common:

(i) The management felt that employee-orientation is necessary for organizational improvement.
(ii) The managers widely shared faith in the capability of employees.
(iii) Active involvement of employees in the programme was considered essential by management.

(iii) *Emphasis on Leader Behaviour*

Leader behaviour is important in any organizational programme. In some situations, however, leader behaviour is regarded as the central feature of HRD initiatives. In the literature this is referred to as transformation leadership. Singh and Bhandarkar (1990) provide detailed studies of leaders who were able to transform their organizations by extraordinary personal involvement. Examples given are that of Russi Modi in TISCO who enthused people at all levels to set high goals of achievement and provided continuing encouragement to achieve results. Similar examples are given of S.V.S. Raghavan at MMTC, Sinha at Western Coalfields at Pench, S.N. Jain at National Fertilizer and S.P. Sharma at IFFCO, Phulpur. In all these examples the transformational leaders are able to create through personal leadership an environment in which employees could improve their capabilities and achieve an impressive growth. Their strategy consisted of enabling employees to do what they are capable of doing by removing obstacles that prevent them from doing their best, and by recognizing their achievements and encouraging them in this direction.

In practical terms, the design of HRD interventions will have to take four aspects into consideration:

1. What managerial practices would create an environment of growth for people in the organization. This refers to creation of HRD environment.
2. What are the organizational imperatives which can best be handled by involvement of people. This refers to identification of organizational priorities.
3. How should HRD interventions be integrated into the work system so that they become an integral part of the work organization. This refers to developing a way of life, a philosophy of working.
4. How should the effectiveness of the programme be measured. This will enable the programme to remain dynamic.

The designer of HRD interventions has to conceptualize the organizational problems and identify what kind of social interventions would help to solve these problems. In most critical areas the intervention strategies will have to initiate simultaneous action at organizational, departmental and individual levels.

The diagnosis of problem and the approach to HRD would have to consider the total enterprise though planning of action may be carried out in appropriate stages. Indeed action to improve all aspects of the organization at one time could, in most cases, be counter-productive.

This does not mean that the overall plan should be frozen because experience of operating the programme may suggest changes that can lead to rethinking about some aspects of the programme. But it is necessary that the initial plan has the perspective of the totality, and different components of the plan should emerge from and fit into the total programme.

Lastly, the implementation strategy would have to be thought through in detail. Understanding of both the concept and the programme by managers in key managerial positions is necessary. A major difficulty in many organizations is that they have a history of confrontation rather than a balanced relationship or a strategy of consensus building. Consensus on the goals of HRD is difficult to develop in some organizations because of mutual suspicion caused by the strategy of confrontation on the part of both the management and the union. At corporate level this aspect will have to receive special attention. The other handicap is that the goals of human development are seen to be abstract and seem unrealistic to many. It is only through experience that conviction in the programme develops. I think an experimental approach is necessary for the programme to mature, and for conviction about it to grow widely among people. The most difficult part of implementation in most organizations is the scepticism that people have about intentions underlying such programmes. These aspects can be handled through a continuous dialogue and discussion. It is, however, necessary to deal with these aspects because change in the minds of men is possible only through questioning.

Different people in the organization would have different concerns. They would have to be identified. Some of the common concerns are likely to be the following:

(i) Need for knowing more about the programme and the rationale.
(ii) Personal anxieties caused by feelings of inadequacy, disbelief, distrust and the like.
(iii) Genuine disagreement with the approach.
(iv) Organizational practices that discourage action.

The implementation strategy would have to identify these and other problem areas and effectively deal with them. It will need patience, understanding and perseverance to manage the programme.

REFERENCES

Bennis, W.G. (1967). Behavioural Sciences Perspective in Organizational Studies, in Srivastava, S. (Ed), *Behavioural Sciences in Management*, Asia, Bombay.

Dayal, I. HRD in Indian Organizations: Current Perspectives and Future Issues, *Vikalpa*, 1989, 14(4): 9-15.

Dayal, I. Constraints of Legislation on Organisational Effectiveness, *Ind. J. Ind. Rel*, 1967, 2(3): 315-332.

Herzberg, F. (1966), *Work and the Nature of Man*, World Publishing, Ohio.

McGregor, D. (1961). *Human Side of Enterprise*, McGraw-Hill, New York.

McGregor, D. (1966). *Leadership and Motivation*, MIT Press, Cambridge.

Roethlisberger, F.J. (1942). *Management and Morale*, Harvard Univ. Press, Cambridge Mass.

Management Journal, 1992, 5(1): 123-143.

Singh P. and Bhandarkar, A. (1990). *Corporate Success and Transformational Leadership*. Wiley Eastern, New Delhi.

Tannenbaum, A. Control of Organisations: Individual Adjustment and Organisational Performance, *Admn. Science Qtly*, 1962, 7(2): 236-257.

Whyte, W.F. (1959). *Man and Organization*, Richard Irwin, Homewood, Ill.

2

CONCEPT OF MAN IN MANAGEMENT*

The concept of man has influenced management practices in organizations. At times the influence on practices is direct and at other times, subtle. This chapter surveys the concept of man in management literature to help managers examine their own beliefs.

An explicit enunciation of the concept of man has been made by social scientists in the post-Hawthorne writings because this concept is central to the development of a theory and practice of administration. In the earlier writings, the concept of man had to be inferred from writings on management. Of these earlier writings, the more important come from practising managers. Taylor, Foyal, Gulick, Sloan and others were concerned basically with improvement in efficiency. The building of a theory of management was incidental to improving efficiency.

It seems that a greater concern for theory building emerges from persons who have dissociated themselves from practice and devoted themselves to study. There are, of course, notable exceptions to this dissociation such as Chester Bernard who was President of Bell Telephone Company of New Jersey. His book, *The Functions of the Executive* (1938) influenced greatly the work of Herbert Simon, James March, Elton Mayo and others.

---

* Reprinted with some revisions from the *Economic & Political Weekly*, Vol. XVI, No. 22, *Review of Management*, 1981, pp. M.81-M.87.

The concept of man in management has been influenced significantly by three considerations. First, the experience of practising managers. Second the experimental, if limited, data from sociological research by early social scientists. Third, the interpretation of cumulative research data from experience and from behavioural scientists moving towards a more complex formulation about the nature of man.

The three identifiable considerations are:

(i) The Rabble Hypothesis
(ii) The Social Man Hypothesis
(iii) The Complex Man Hypothesis

While none of these concepts is exclusive, the implications of each of them for management's theory of man are interesting and important.

(i) The Rabble Hypothesis

It assumes man's nature to be inert, that he must have things done for him. The major contributions to this view have been made by economists and technicians who regarded man as an instrument for action rather than the central figure who makes the choice for action. His support is to be obtained by giving him attractive incentives. He is to be moulded to achieve the goals of his superior(s).

Analysing the work of Ricardo, the economist, Mayo (1949, p. 37) suggests that Ricardo bases his studies and his logic on the following three concepts:

(i) Natural society consists of a horde of unorganized individuals.
(ii) Every individual acts in a manner calculated to secure his self-preservation or self-interest.

(iii) Every individual thinks logically, to the best of his ability, in the service of his aim.

Those assumptions characterize many earlier theorists up to World War II. Implied in the rabble hypothesis "is the conviction of need for Leviathan, a powerful State, which by the exercise of a unique authority shall impose order on the rabble" [Mayo, 1949, p. 40]. For management, the implications of this hypothesis was that the work of employees had to be arranged to serve the goals of the organization either by coercion or extra inducement. This approach is widely shared by some of the most significant writings in the 1920s and 1930s.

Frederick Taylor, who is regarded as the father of scientific management, makes three propositions:

(i) Functional specification and prescribing the best way of doing work;
(ii) Functional supervision;
(iii) Incentive to worker to work beyond the prescribed norm.

Describing the essential features of his scientific management, Taylor writes (1947, p. 39):

> "Perhaps the most prominent single element in modern scientific management is the task idea. The work of every workman is fully planned by the management at least one day in advance, and each man receives in most cases complete written instructions, describing in detail the task which he is to accomplish, as well as the means to be used in doing the work." Further, he says, "And whenever the workman succeeds in doing his task right, and within the time limit specified, he receives an addition of

from 30 to 100 per cent to his ordinary wages."

Max Weber famed for having developed the concept of bureaucracy, was also influenced by his direct contact with work and his observation of arbitrariness in the management of organizations. He felt that some order and rationality in the work system was needed. He set out a series of propositions for the creation of a legal-rational system although he was much later appalled by some of the consequences of his system on human organization.

While Weber sought to protect people from arbitrary action, he proposed the principle of legitimizing authority and emphasized the importance and form of a position. The person holding it may change but the job's form and content may not. Work is organized into functional divisions; so is supervision, thus creating functional command. Depersonalization is emphasized by selection and recruitment being assigned to an independent authority. The machine-like precision Weber sought to attain in the organization had other limitations that would become massive with time; delays, a premium on mediocrity, a neglect of innovation, causing serious problems in the co-ordination of work because functional departments develop thick impenetrable walls around them (Gouldner, 1955; Merton, 1952; Blau, 1955), and so on.

In Weber's formulations, as in Taylor's, the employee is the recipient: He needs to receive direction from his superior; to have his work planned by his superior and he must achieve for his superior what the superior specifies.

Briefly, the characteristics of man in the Rabble Hypothesis are the following:

(i) Man is disorganized and works primarily for his personal ends.
(ii) Given adequate incentive he could be made to do

what the manager desires of him.

It is clear how this concept of man has come to be variously described as the economic man or the machine man.

Herzberg gives an interesting biblical description to this concept by naming it the Adam concept of man and differentiating it from the Abraham concept. Herzberg (1966) says:

> "The first definition of man is the creation of Adam. Adam was created as the perfect man, *albeit* "feebleminded" because he was created without knowledge. "And the Lord God commanded the man, saying, of every tree of the garden thou mayest eat, but of the tree of knowledge of good and evil, thou shall not eat of it; for in the day that thou eatest thereof thou shall surely die." (*Genesis* 2: 16; p. 15).

The other view of man's nature appeared in the conversation between God and Abraham:

> "And when Abraham was ninety years old and nine, the Lord appeared to Abraham, and said unto him: I am God Almighty; walk before Me, and be thou whole hearted, and I will make My covenant between Me and thee and will multiply thee exceedingly.... And thou shall be the father of a multitude of nations." (*Genesis* 12:1; p 15).

Implication for Management

The Rabble Hypothesis implies that (a) two distinct entities exist in an organization, one concerned with *doing*, the other with *determining* what is best for the man and the organization; and (b) the manager must plan and organize the doer's behaviour for achieving the mission of the organization.

It is not surprising that large-scale expression of these views has been found on the organization of work; fragmentation of tasks, determination of standard procedures of work, incentive payment. In fairness to Taylor, these practices were only a part of the concepts that he and his colleagues had formulated. In practice, the implementation became partial, lacking the sharing of responsibility on which he laid so much emphasis.

If we examine the way organizations function, and take a close look at the patterns of leadership behaviour in organisations, it is not difficult to see that the Rabble Hypothesis, more than any other, is generally accepted among the managerial ranks in India and other developing countries, even though the statements made of the concept of man may be greatly different.

(ii) **The Social Man Hypothesis**

The now classic experiments in the Hawthorne plant of Western Electric near Chicago, pioneered by Elton Mayo and F.J. Roethlisberger of Harvard University created a trend in thinking that led to the social man hypothesis. The series of Relay Assembly Test Room experiments made the startling revelation that changes in physical conditions of work influenced performance less than the experience of being recognized as important. When the experimental conditions of work such as lighting, rest pauses, canteen facilities, physical comfort, etc., were withdrawn in the last round of experimental changes in the Relay Assembly Test Room, the experimenters found that the productivity went up instead of going down (Roethlisberger and Dickson, 1939). The Bank Wiring Observation Room experiments provided invaluable knowledge of the dynamics of group work. They revealed the process of socialization, how members become a cohesive group, how they acquire social status, how leadership emerges and how reward and punishment for defiant behaviour are practised for the maintenance of the group's norms, etc. The experiments on group behaviour at Hawthorne initiated a large number of experiments on group dynamics [Cartwright and Zander, 1962; Homans, 1950]. They threw up significant facts. Groups exercise a powerful influence on the behaviour of an individual, and this influence in some cases is pervasive. If the status on differential basis of skill classification or hierarchy drawn up by management differs from what has been determined by the group, the group's norms and values prevail over that of the management. The sentiments of the group members for one another were more important than the differential work status as laid down by management in setting up wage levels, or the hierarchy. The study of group behaviour has been an extremely well-researched field since the Bank Wiring Observation Room and most of the findings of Howthorne studies have been confirmed in subsequent research studies.

Roethlisberger (1942, pp. 20-21) states the essence of the thesis of the social man hypothesis thus:

> "It will be remembered that at first the investigators assumed a simple and direct relation between certain physical changes in the worker's environment and his responses to them. This simple and direct relation is illustrated in Diagram 1. But all the evidence of the early experiments showed that the responses of employees to changes in their immediate working environment can be understood only in terms of their attitudes — the 'meaning' these changes have for them. The point of view is represented in Diagram 2. However, the 'meaning' which these changes have for the worker is not strictly and primarily logical, for

they are fraught with human feelings and values. . . ." And further "Sentiments do not appear in a vacuum; they do not come out of the blue; they appear in a social context, and apart from it they are likely to be misunderstood."

The 'meaning', therefore, which any individual worker assigns to a particular change depends upon:

(1) his social 'conditioning', or what sentiments (values, hopes, fears, expectations, etc.) he is bringing to the work situation because of his previous family and group associations, and hence the relation of the change to these sentiments; and
(2) the kind of human satisfaction he is deriving from his social participation with other workers and supervisors in the immediate work group of which he is a member, and hence the effect of the change on his customary interpersonal relations.

Diagram 1

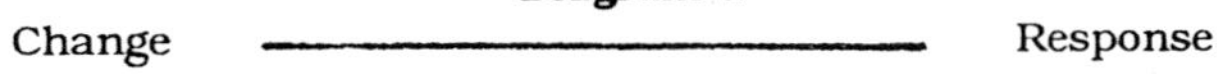

Diagram 2

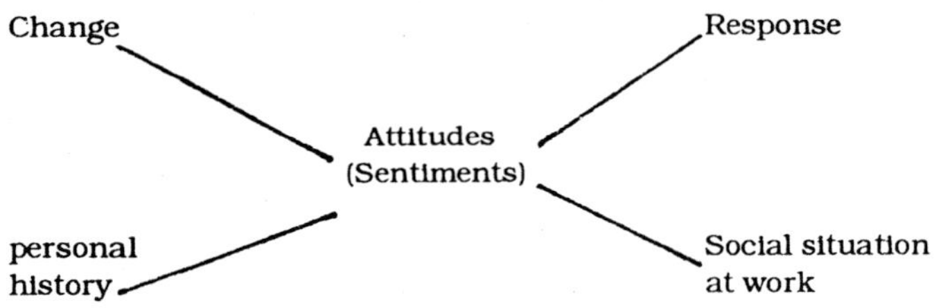

The Hawthorne Studies began in the mid-20s and a great many writings in the late 30s and 40s, and even later, were influenced by the findings of these studies.

In protest of the writings of the scientific school of

Taylor and his colleagues, Mayo and others were raising serious questions about the seamy side of industrial progress, its impact on the people who were fast becoming alien to the fragmented work that industry demanded of them. While recognizing the material advantages of industrial advancement, social scientists have been greatly concerned about the danger spots that industrial society harboured, with its potential for destroying historical, social and personal relationships (Durkheim, 1952; Casson, 1973).

The humanists among social scientists seriously questioned the economic man concept, depicting man as striving mainly to serve his own ends, spurred on by financial incentives. The findings of Hawthorne and subsequent studies lifted the curtain on affiliative and social membership motives, showing them up as being as powerful as the economic, and sometimes even more. They suggested that man lived not by bread alone: recognition, belonging and sentiments were powerful motives for his behaviour at work.

The humanist concern assumes the individual as capable of exercising a relatively high degree of imagination, ingenuity, creativity at his work, and of learning to accept responsibility if the conditions are conducive. McGregor (1960) has distinguished sharply between the traditional assumptions about man which he labels Theory X and the research-based assumptions he made, naming them Theory Y. The traditional assumptions regard man as having an innate dislike of work and will avoid it if he can. He prefers to be directed, and will avoid responsibility, if he can. He has to be, therefore, closely supervised, and given external inducements to work.

Theory Y states that, given the appropriate conditions, man seeks out responsibility, takes the initiative and the risk if his work needs them; that man is self-directing and result achieving if his work satisfies his other needs. The supervisor's concern assumes the responsibility for creating conditions in which man can satisfy his self-actualization needs.

The social man hypothesis advocates the recognition of the significance of his being a member of his social group and having distinctive motives, sentiments and feelings. Man's response to external stimuli would have to relate to his individual identity. The supervisor's bidding would be followed fully or partially depending on how the employee feels about him. Thus, Roethlisberger writes (1942, p. 9):

> "It is my simple thesis that a human problem requires a human solution. First, we have to learn to recognize a human problem when we see one: and, second, upon recognizing it, we have to learn to deal with it as such and not as if it were something else. Too often, at the verbal level, we talk glibly about the importance of the human factor; and too seldom at the concrete level of behaviour do we recognize a human problem for what it is and deal with it as such. A human problem to be brought to a human solution requires human data and human tools."

The humanistic orientation was an aspect of changes that were taking place in society due to rapid industrial growth and the growing concern for a democratic social order in several countries in the West. The industrial society had ushered in major changes in relation to man such as displacement of human skills by the machine and the fragmentation and routinization of operations at the shop floor and at clerical levels (Friedman, 1955; Walker, 1962). Observers of the industrial society were concerned over man's alienation from his work, and the control that the machine was exercising over man. The social scientists showed concern not only for these aspects but also over the effect of the stresses and strains of industrial work on mental health of employees (Mayo, 1949).

Of the social man hypothesis, the implications for management were:

(a) The supervisor must understand the sentiments and feelings of employees because this understanding would induce more satisfaction and better performance. The most important task of the supervisor is to create conditions in which the employee could do his best;

(b) the social system of work organization is as important as the technical: the recognition of it is essential for effective management.

Implications for Management

In industry, the practical manifestations of the social man hypothesis emerged in the shape of a great many welfare programmes ranging from counselling of employees as in the Hawthorne plant, to the establishing of subsidized canteens, home visits, health programmes, recreation, etc. It was assumed that "by being human", the supervisor would create the environment suitable for work. Some organizations initiated welfare schemes that took care of them from birth to the tomb and gave rise to the expression "welfared to death" and in some cases, "the country club management".

(iii) **The Complex Man Hypothesis**

The continuing involvement of scientists from several social science disciplines in the study of management has contributed to the complex man hypothesis. Man's behaviour is subject to his particular situation of work, the nature of interpersonal and intergroup relations, and to his individual, personal history. A new concept of man emerges from an increased knowledge of his complex and shifting needs, a concept that nudged out the oversimplified, innocent, push-button idea of inert man.

The behavioural data that go to formulate the complex man hypothesis come from different sources. Bennis writes (1966, p. 187):

- From psychology we have psychoanalytic role, and cognitive theories;
- From sociology there are bureaucratic, social-system, symbolic interactionism, and role theories;
- From anthropology have sprung the central ideas of norms, sentiments, cohesion and interaction;
- From political science has come the recent work on conflict theory;
- From economics the decision processes and choice mechanisms have been elucidated;
- From the historical approach have come mainly case studies which have helped to clarify the role of key decision-makers.

As in the social man hypothesis, man is seen to be propelled by his inner motives. But the motives are varied and the response pattern, complex. Through interactions with people in childhood and from experiences of pain and pleasure, the individual acquires a set of attitudes and values and a perception of external reality which forms his private and personal world. His world is a complex one, for he is conscious of some motives and blind to others. He has explanations for some reactions to people and situations, none for others. As an adult, conscious and unconscious motives influence his responses to work and to people. He adjusts to some situations more easily than to others; in a given situation he can establish positive relations with some and not with others. His reactions, or behavioural responses, are dependent upon and are modified by a large variety of interactions with other people and what he learns from a variety of experiences in his life. Notwithstanding such differences, there is consistency in the individual's response to similar situations. Children from domineering parents respond to authority either by submission or by rejection; whatever the response, the individual would continue to react to authority in his characteristic way. Some individuals cannot distinguish one type of authority from another, family, social or work situations. Their characteristic response to authority in family, for example, extends to their relation and response with the supervisor at work. The concept of complex man suggests that:

(1) An individual's response to work situation is guided by his history and the experience he has with people and situations in his environment.

(2) All actions are not known to the individual because he is unconscious of some motives of behaviour. Understanding the cause and effect (or stimulus-response) relationship in individual and group behaviour requires greater knowledge of unconscious and semi-conscious motives. On the whole, however, there is consistency in the individual's response to the same kind of stimuli, and situations.

(3) The individual's behaviour is directed from within – by his own personality predispositions – but he is influenced significantly by his continuing experiences and the interactions in his environment. Learning from a given situation depends upon the individual himself, with the capability varying one from the other.

Implications for Management

The managerial implications of the complex man hypothesis are many. The manager's awareness and his capacity to recognize individual differences in his relationship with people assume great importance. He must strive to develop positive relationships with subordinates, peers and superiors by understanding the characteristics of both individual and group behaviour. There is no single measure on the part of management that can motivate all people at all times to work for organizational goals.

Because several aspects of the environment influence behaviour, the management need to act in several ways to induce the desired patterns of behaviour. The pattern of interactions at work, the styles of leadership and the situation greatly play upon man's behaviour at work (Dayal, 1976). The first two aspects have long been a subject of study; the impact of the work situation has been studied extensively during the past 20/25 years. Indeed, there are many research findings to support the thesis that the nature of work (work technology) influence behaviour of people at work (Whyte, 1969, Dubin, 1965). Likewise, people respond differently to controls (Tennenbaum, 1962; Wood ward, 1970) and to policies and practices in organizations (Merton, 1952; Mouzelis, 1967).

Given the complexity of behaviour, the manager requires the skills of understanding *how* man behaves – the process – and not only the skills of knowing *what* needs to be done – the content. He must have as great an understanding of how a policy should be implemented as the substantive nature of the policy itself. From the complex man hypothesis, the prescriptions for management are likely to include:

(a) leadership that is capable of analysing the patterns in human situations;
(b) development of an appropriate work organization, i.e., design that allows both task and social relationships to develop; and
(c) policies and practices which support rather than hinder performance and relationships at work.

Three Approaches Compared

The notions about the concept of man in management are derived from the data obtained in research, from the observations and experience of the manager and the theorist. The predispositions of the manager and the theorist and the context in which they study their primary data have influenced their concept of man. The social environment of the theorist, the values and attitudes of the community, and the nature of the behavioural data have all exerted their influence. Taylor's concern for efficiency and the values and attitudes about man in his social environment were as significant as the objective data he may have used for formulating his concept. The humanist concern in the social man hypothesis has likewise been influenced by the general environment of the period.

The Rabble Hypothesis conceives man as being amenable to doing what his superior tells him to do. So long as he is compensated, he would do what he is required to do, as does a machine. The Social Man Hypothesis postulates that the individual would strive toward satisfying his needs and sentiments. He would work towards achieving organizational goals if he *felt* that the supervisor recognized these feelings, and there was an equation between what is needed by him and what the organization provides.

The Complex Man Hypothesis views him as the

initiator, one who responds to the external stimuli according to his own history and background. It emphasizes that man is inner-directed and self-motivating. This concept has evolved from behavioural studies while trying to explain and predict behaviour. The Freudian concept of the *unconscious self* has been an important contributor to this formulation. In practice, however, this concept is generally accepted at cognitive level but has not been used widely in either policy formulation or managerial practices.

Current Status

McGregor (1960, 1966) has said that the manager's assumptions about man will decide how he will manage people. Underlying his strategy for action is the assumption he makes about what motivates the employee. In spite of the theoretical or research-based ideas about the nature of man, a manager is guided by his own experiences and comes to conclusions about the *nature of man* from these experiences. The concept of man so developed is used by him in formulating his own style of dealing with other people, and in developing his administrative strategy. At the core of his administrative policy is a manager's concept of man; In exploring the concept, two considerations deserve attention:

(1) It is generally mentioned in organizations that if the supervisor is *human* or *close* to his subordinates, they take advantage of the relationship and neglect work. Hence, the supervisor would do well to maintain a distance from them. This impression may be based on partial or selective data; but it still guides man's impressions of man. We would have to draw upon much more varied data from wide sources to guide

our conclusions.

(2) The application of the Complex Man Hypothesis to management requires much understanding of human behaviour, the sensitivity to appreciate it. There are no ready-made prescriptions of how the superior should relate to people, nor are they even possible. The administrator must have an understanding of the motives of his own behaviour and of the behaviour of other people with whom he interacts. He must know why he reacts favourably to some and not to others; why some people respond to him warmly and others are hostile or indifferent; why is the same person responsive in some matters and not in others. The administrator must know and feel what influence the system has on the human organization and on the patterns of relationships, and how he would have to take the totality of the behavioural and organizational factors for choosing a particular course of action. The assumptions of the complex man hypothesis would need different kinds of approaches to administration than do the simpler formulations of the rabble hypothesis.

At the work place where events take place in quick succession, and pressures for results are constantly exerted, supervisors often find short term solutions to deal with immediate problems. Over time these solutions themselves become problems. Let me take an example to illustrate the point. An employee gives below average output inspite of friendly coaxing by the supervisor, but improves his output only when threatened by a show cause notice. A few experiences, of this kind lead to the conclusion that tough handling is needed to get work out of the employee. These conclusions are further reinforced by similar experiences of his peers. When this approach is used widely by supervisors in the work place, employees develop counter-coercise strategies such as producing lower quality material, fudging data, and alignment with aggressive trade unions, etc. The stage is set for a confrontation strategy in dealing with people in the organization. Any amount of discussion on alternative motivational strategies to improve output would seem unrealistic. Basically, assumptions about people are derived from the reaction to the action taken by the manager to find an immediate solution to his work related problems, without sufficient consideration of alternative approaches to solving the problems at hand. Inadvertently images about people, and relationships are built up in the mind of the manager. These images take a firm shape over time and guide his administrative action.

Notwithstanding the problems, there is greater realization, at least at the overt level, that real-life situations are complex and that simple formulations about the behaviour of people yield poor results. Failures often reveal to the more perceptive among us the need to re-examine the living reality. This step is surely the beginning of the acceptance of complex models of action. I believe that the change in our perceptions of man in live situations would have to go through this process of learning through failures before we arrive at a concept of the working man that is at once dynamic and true.

REFERENCES

Barnard, C. (1938). *The Functions of the Executive*, Harvard University Press, Cambridge, Massachusetts.

Bennis, W.G. (1966). *Leadership and Motivation*, MIT Press, Cambridge, Massachusetts.

Blau, P. (1955). *The Dynamics of Bureaucratic Structure: A Study of Interpersonal Relations in Two Government Agencies*, University of Chicago Press, Chicago, Illinois.

Cartwright, D. and Zander, A. (1962). *Group Dynamics*, Row, Peterson, Illinois.

Casson, Stanley (1937). *Progress and Catastrophe*, Harper, New York.

Dayal, I. (1976). *Designing a Work Organisation*, All India Management

Association, New Delhi.

Dubin, R. (1965), *Supervision and Productivity: Emprical Findings and Theoretical Considerations, in Leadership and Productivity*, Chandler, San Francisco.

Durkheim, Emile (1952). *Suicide: A Study in Sociology*, Routledge and Kegan Paul, London.

Friedman, G. (1955). *Industrial Society*, The Free Press of Glencoe, Illinois.

Gouldner, A. (1955). *Patterns of Industrial Bureaucracy*, Routledge and Kegan Paul, London.

Herzberg, F. (1966). *Work and the Nature of Man*, World Publishing, Ohio.

Homans, G. (1950). *The Human Group*, Harcourt, Brace, New York.

Mayo, E. (1949). *The Social Problems of an Industrial Civilisation*, Routledge and Kegan Paul, London.

McGregor, D. (1966). *Leadership and Motivation*, MIT Press, Cambridge, Massachusetts.

Merton, R. (1952). *Bureaucratic Structure and Personality*, in *Reader in Bureaucracy*, Free Press of Glencoe, Illinois.

Mouzelis, N.P. (1967). *Organisation and Bureaucracy*, Routledge and Kegan Paul, London.

Rice, A.K. (1958). *Productivity and Social Organisation*, Tavistock, London.

Roethlisberger, F.J. (1968) *Man-in-Organisation*, The Belknap Press of Harvard University Press, Cambridge, Massachusetts.

Roethlisberger, F.J. (1942). *Management and Morale*, Harvard University Press, Cambridge, Massachusetts.

Roethlisberger, F.J. and Dickson, W.T. (1939). *Management and the Worker*, Harvard University Press, Cambridge, Massachusetts.

Tannenbaum, A. Control in Organisation: "Individual Adjustment and Organisational Performance", *Admin. Sc., Qly.*, 1962, 7(2): 236-257.

Taylor, F.W. (1911). *Scientific Management*, Harper, New York.

Taylor, F.W. (1947). *Principles of Scientific Management*, Harper, New York.

Trist, E.L. and Bamforth, K.W. *Some Social and Psychological Consequences of the Longwall Method of Coal Geeting, Human Relations"*, 1951, 4: 3-38.

Walker, C. (1962). *Modern Civilisation and Technology"*, McGraw-Hill, New York.

Weber, Max (1947). *The Theory of Social and Economic Organisations*, The Free Press of Glencoe, Illinois.

Whyte, W.F. (1959). *Man and Organisation*, Richard Irwin, Homewood, Illinois.

Woodward, J. (Ed) (1970). *Organisation and Productivity*, Oxford University Press, London.

3

HRD IN INDIAN ORGANIZATIONS: Current Perspectives and Future Issues*

In recent years, HRD has emerged as a distinct area of concern in organizations. This paper presents an overview of HRD practices in a variety of Indian organizations and identifies areas that need attention of HRD managers and academicians.

There are three distinctly identifiable approaches among Indian organizations that have formal HRD programmes: (a) Man-Centred Approach, (b) Reciprocal Approach, and (c) Selective Approach. Although in practice there are overlaps among these approaches, this classification is useful for discussing the various patterns of HRD initiatives.

Man-Centred Approach

Based on humanistic considerations, HRD, according to this approach, is a philosophy shared by organizations that believe development of people to be their primary responsibility. This belief governs personnel, welfare, and other organizational policies and practices concerning its employees. Factors such as promoting trust, open communication, authenticity in interpersonal relation-

* Revised. Original published in Vol. 14, No. 4, Oct.-Dec. 1989 issue of *Vikalpa — The Journal for Decision Makers*, Published by the Indian Institute of Management, Ahmedabad. Reproduced with permission.

ships, and welfare of employees and their families are given top priority. Development of people thus becomes an end in itself in such organizations.

The assumption underlying this approach is that improving an employee's capability and developing him/her is the responsibility of the employer and, therefore, should be pursued as a programme. This style of management favours personalized relationships. It is more likely to be found in family-managed organizations than in those managed by paid chief executives. Such organizations have progressive welfare practices for employees and their families and a managerial orientation which can be described as paternal. They follow practices that are way beyond what is required by law with respect to matters like health, education, housing, retirement benefits and canteen facilities. J.N. Tata, Shri Ram, Walchand Hirachand, T.V. Sundaram Iyengar and a few other industrialists started welfare practices much before legislation on these matters was even framed. This approach emphasizes the salience of extrinsic job factors. Management-employee relationships are generally informal. The senior management staff attend to the well-being of employees at all levels. Trust and confidence between employees and employer are built through personalized relationships. This often enables managers to practise openness in their relationships. The most important feature in such organizations is the confidence the employees have in the chief executive. He is a father figure and is respected by employees at all levels. Some typical examples from companies that have followed this style of management are given below:

- After a prolonged discussion with the General Manager of a company regarding punishment meted out to some employees, the union leaders requested the chief executive to intervene and told him that his decision in the matter would be accepted by everyone. The chief executive was considered by employees as being impartial and one who would be fair to all. He was not perceived as fitting into the managerial hierarchy.

- The chief executive of an organization was away for about six months on an assignment. The employees felt that they owed it to the "head of the family" to keep peace in the organization while he was away. On his return, however, the employees were anxious to know whether he would come back to the company and give it the same attention he had given earlier as various problems that could threaten the harmony of the organization had developed in his absence.
- When a company was doing poorly, a large number of employees offered to accept a cut in their salaries until profits improved. Accordingly, their salaries were cut and were restored only when the company's fortunes improved. The chief executive did not draw any salary during this period.
- The chief executive of a company believed that poor financial performance of the company was due to inadequate planning, poor assessment of market demand, and failure to improve production technology for which, however, higher management was responsible. Therefore, he decided that workers should not be denied their bonus if they had worked as hard as they did in the previous years.

Organizational Characteristics

The organizations that successfully use the Man-centred Approach consciously follow certain methods of developing managers who would preserve the system. Some common features of these organizations include:

Building a Coterie

The chief executive develops a group of people around him who are totally loyal to him and who are included in private discussions. The approach adopted by Shri Ram of DCM is a case in point. An examination of Shri Ram's biography and the private correspondence between him and his general managers at Jay Engineering Works shows how these loyal persons were sent to various units of the organization and groomed for their positions. Shri Ram would also discuss various matters of the company with his general managers at early morning walks or at meals. The managers were given opportunities to observe Shri Ram in his business and social interactions. They could thus learn his style of managing company affairs (Dayal, Srivastava and Alfred, 1972). The company also recruited many people as apprentices and the best among them were picked out by the leader for key positions in the organization. Once an employee became a member of the coterie, he was treated more like a family member and less like an employee.

Visibility

The leader is visible. He takes regular rounds at the factory and meets a large number of people during the course of each day. For instance, the General Manager of Jay Engineering Works, T.R. Gupta who was groomed by Shri Ram knew most of the 2,500 employees by name and visited their houses on festivals and other special occasions.

Autonomy

The general manager is not required to explain his actions. There is little interference with his plans and decisions. He is encouraged to feel more like an owner and less like an employee in the organization. In turn, he develops more managers in the pattern set by his mentors. For example, in his personal letters to T.R. Gupta, Shri Ram repeatedly asked him to take necessary decisions himself as he was on the site and knew the situation best. Mandelia, chief executive of the successful Birla enterprise, has stated that apart from sending periodic reports to the headquarters, he was totally free to manage the plant.

Symbolic Gestures

Symbolic gestures indicative of family-like relationships are built into the social system of the organization. Organizations evolve unique patterns to emphasize this aspect. Shri Ram, for example, made it a point to celebrate *Holi* with his employees every year because it is an important festival for them. The organization also arranged *Ram Lila* celebrations every year where attendance was compulsory. The chief executive of the TVS group invites the family members of employees to visit the factory on special occasions. The employees are also given food packets to take home. These ritualistic gestures help to reinforce family-like affiliations and paternal styles of relationships in organizations.

Welfare Activities

Many welfare measures for employees and their families are instituted by some organizations. In most cases, these measures are way ahead of the legal provisions in such matters. For example, companies like Tata, DCM, TVS and Kirloskar have been pioneers in introducing many measures for the security and well-being of their employees and their families.

HRD Philosophy

The patterns of relationships at work reflect the HRD philosophy. In some organizations, the practices and philosophy of HRD are perpetuated by the managers who are encouraged to follow the role model of their seniors. In the process of organizational socialization, they internalize the values and attitudes of their leaders. The entire process is thus institutionalized. This is somewhat akin to the kind of "apprenticeship" prevailing in Japanese organizations to prepare young persons for positions of responsibility.

Problems

The first and perhaps the most important difficulty with this approach relates to leadership change in the organization. The strength of such organizations lies in the special relationship built by people at the top with their subordinates. When there is a change in leadership, realignment in relationships has to take place. If the succeeding leader does not believe in this style of management or does not recognize its relevance or virtue, the relationships of trust are rarely sustained. For instance, when Lala Charat Ram succeeded his father as chairman of Jay Engineering Works, the organization went through a long period of adjustment as he had a very different style of leadership (Dayal, Srivastava and Alfred, 1972).

The second difficulty arises when there is a change in technology. The new technology may require a high level of technical knowledge rather than experience, and this may necessitate changes in recruitment practices, work flow relationships, and in the existing social hierarchy. With the introduction of computers, the accountant is no longer the sole repository of financial information as he was in the earlier system. Some family-managed organizations have handled these problems effectively. In Sundaram Clayton, for instance, promotions are now given on merit and not on seniority.

The third difficulty arises due to changes in the aspirations of the young. The youth in general today want more individual recognition and independence and do not like social differentiation and stratification. They are on the whole less comfortable with paternal styles that create dependency and prevent development of an independent identity. These attitudes and personal values often cause conflicts in organizations based on paternal styles of management.

Reciprocal Approach

This perspective comes partly from humanistic and partly from business interests. It regards development of people as the most important asset for either improving or sustaining organizational performance. The emphasis of the HRD programme here is on developing roles, role relationships, appraisal systems, training, job design, etc. In some cases, most of the traditional personnel functions are included in the HRD system. This approach assumes that HRD is important for growth of the organization. Since growth of an organization is linked to growth of people, it is in the interest of the organization to develop human resources.

In general, organizations take up HRD at times of diversification, intensive growth and declining profits. The HRD strategy and the focus of the programme are broadly linked to the circumstance of the enterprise. Some examples are given below:

- ITC took up HRD at the time of diversifying its business from cigarette manufacturing to other products. The company concentrated on improving its appraisal system and providing training so as to identify and rapidly develop managers for new projects.

- Crompton Greaves resorted to HRD when it faced a slump in business and decided to take up additional projects in new locations. The focus of its programme was role clarity so that responsibility for results could be vested with profit centre managers. It refined the appraisal system as well.
- The HRD programme at L&T was associated with its programme of organizational development.
- The programme at SBI centred around training and appraisal following its reorganization and rapid growth (Silvera, 1988; Rao et al., 1988; Rao and Pereira, 1986).
- HRD in LIC followed its reorganization and sustained growth.

These examples show that HRD in most organizations is part of an overall strategy for improving its performance; it is not an isolated programme. L&T, SBI, LIC, ITC and many others took up comprehensive programmes for reorganizing, reorienting corporate activities, prior to or simultaneously with their HRD programme.

Organizational Features

The practices followed by organizations for growth of individuals differ considerably. They range from job redesign, e.g. Bharat Heavy Engineering Corporation where responsibility for planning and results now rests with the employees on the shop floor, to counselling, job rotation, training and the like. Both in focus and variety, HRD in each organization is designed to serve its own needs and follows an approach that is unique.

Some HRD practitioners have developed HRD systems which include mainly functions that earlier well-developed personnel departments carried out in organizations (Strauss and Sayles, 1985; Pigors, Myers and Malm, 1959; Athreya, 1988). Athreya suggests that an HRD consists of the following 12 elements (p. 380): Corporate Planning; Manpower Forecasting, Selection, Induction and Placement; Role Analysis; Appraisal; Counselling; Self-development; Career Planning; Succession Planning; Job Rotation; Training; and Data Bank. It is assumed that these functions will be carried out with a developmental orientation and will have a sharper humanistic perspective.

A review of HRD programmes in organizations suggest that three distinct features differentiate HRD from traditional personnel management:

> The growth of the individual as a total human being is seen to be the most important aim of an HRD programme. In whatever activity the organization may be involved, one significant output should be growth and development of individuals who are engaged in that activity. Therefore, involvement, exercise of discretion in performing the job, autonomy, job design, etc. become areas of concern for HRD programmes.
>
> The individual is seen to be a total person and not an employee in an assigned job. Hence, development of individual's total capabilities, and not skill alone, assumes importance in HRD initiatives.
>
> The growth of the organization must form an integral part of an HRD programme. Growth of individuals without that of the organization is not sustainable. Hence, the HRD programme should aim at development of the system as a whole. In this respect, organizational analysis often becomes an important concern for the management. Hence, a programme with individual growth as the objective and linkages that enable and sustain organizational

growth are necessary.

Processes Involved

Several studies show that growth occurs when an individual is able to acquire new perspectives about his work, the job, the environment, and relationships. Often the individual gains fresh understanding of his job when he assesses his particular contribution; he also gains new insights through interactions with other people. Four conditions are required for fostering individual growth:

- personal desire to grow
- experiencing a wide range of interactions with people and the environment
- assimilating this experience to derive a new meaning of things, relationships and situations
- assessing the results with a view to knowing one's ability/potential and using this in planning future action.

Briefly, a concern for development must be generated from within. The individual should be able to identify his strengths and weaknesses, his needs for learning, and how he could improve his capabilities. The organization would have to provide scope for learning; the job should enable an individual to experiment with new skills, relationships at work, and an opportunity to assess his strengths and weaknesses. While the individual would have to assume responsibility for his growth, the work organization would have to be flexible enough to respond to the individual's growth needs. This requirement also suggests that the HRD programme will be less effective if opportunities to arrange work flexibly are unavailable. For example, it should be possible to redesign work on the shopfloor for some persons, even if such changes are not made for all.

In Glacier studies, Brown and Jaques (1965) developed the rationale of work organization before undertaking specific programmes of interpersonal relationships. The work organization covered identification of roles, role relationships, representative and executive systems, policy framework to guide all aspects of work activity and the like. They felt that a rational work organization is necessary before taking up an intervention programme to develop human relationships. The two cannot be separated. This point is important while developing HRD.

Another aspect that contributes to work culture is the design of work organization. It should give the employee control over such aspects of work as influence results. In such a system, inter-departmental cooperation also becomes easier. If a person has to constantly depend upon other units, as on a conveyor belt, he becomes dependent upon others for results. The socio-technical systems developed during the past 30 years have been extensively used in the organization of work (Rice, 1958; Trist et al., 1963; Dayal and Dayal, 1983). Socio-technical concepts were used in the reorganization of BHEL, SBI, LIC and others.

The initiative for self-development would, therefore, depend upon several things, the most important among them being:

- The explicitness of the social organization, work roles, the patterns of interaction among its members and the values and attitudes that the organization represents.
- The cooperation among people and achievement of results that the design of the work organization promotes.
- The decision-making and problem-solving systems through which the management conveys its concern for human growth to individuals.

Selective Approach

The third approach is succession planning which has been practised for many years by personnel departments in a number of organizations. It consists of identifying promising persons and carefully grooming them for leadership positions. Generally such programmes apply to senior and middle level managers and not to employees as a whole. The important elements of this approach consist of skills in identifying promising persons and developing special programmes such as assignments, placement in select positions, training and the like. Being selective, this approach does not strictly fit the definition of HRD discussed earlier in this chapter.

HRD Perspective

The HRD approach has philosophical underpinnings – it encompasses employees as a whole and does not confine itself to development of managerial manpower or succession planning. The HRD perspective has to examine intrinsic besides extrinsic factors for human satisfaction (McGregor, 1966). In this sense, HRD approaches come close to the concerns of programmes on quality of work life (Davis and Cherms, 1975; De, 1984). The HRD programmes include initiatives for growth and satisfaction of employees at all levels, redesign of work, discretionary component in the job, and autonomy. Hence, HRD has three related aspects:

- Widely shared belief by the management in developing the individual and the desire to convert this philosophy into a strategy.
- Link between the work organization and individual plan for development and encouraging flexibility in the administrative organization.
- Several programmes to improve organizational

performance.

HRD is not an isolated exercise. Organizational development or other programmes are invariably taken up with it. The interdependence between individual growth and work roles is not noticed in many HRD programmes. The programme to rationalize the work organization has, in many cases, preceded HRD. This has been observed with regard to SBI, LIC, Crompton Greaves, Bank of Baroda, IOCL and others.

Future Directions

HRD deserves increased attention of both managers and the academicians. HRD in organizations is necessary for effectively coping with changes in the environment, expectations of the new breed of employees, and the need for adjustment to rapid changes in technology. Sustained leadership of organizations is likely to depend on the success of their HRD programmes.

HRD is also important in the societal context. Lack of development at work is reflected in unsatisfactory relationships in the family and society. Alienation at work contributes to growing discontent among the young and a feeling of anger for established institutions, Positive experiences at work are necessary for developing collaborative societal relationships.

Areas of Concern

Considering the importance of HRD for organizations, it is necessary to identify the areas or issues that need examination. Some of these are identified here:

1. What is the difference between traditional personnel functions and HRD? If HRD is merely a change in terminology, the position should be

clearly stated. If the two are different, the distinction should be highlighted. Experience shows that even when HRD philosophical reorientation is given to traditional personnel functions, they do not, on their own, lead to development of individuals.

An attempt has been made in this chapter to draw the difference between HRD and the traditional personnel functions. I hold the view that HRD will have a greater impact on organizations if it is distinguished from personnel functions. This view is based on the premise that HRD has to be action-oriented and rooted in the problem areas. The scope of HRD is wide and it would be more effective if it is a separate function. The decision to set up HRD as a separate unit will depend primarily on how the programme is conceived and the purpose it is meant to serve.

2. Is HRD dependent upon OD? If they are linked, should they be handled simultaneously or sequentially? Would HRD have less impact if it is not linked to OD? From the literature on HRD, the difference between HRD and OD is not clear (National HRD Network Papers, 1989).
3. How should operators in routine tasks such as clerical employees be involved in HRD? Does the nature of their work contain intrinsic motivational factors? Job redesign has been attempted in some places but the exercise is difficult and time consuming. It is unlikely that large organizations will frequently undertake a job redesign exercise. What are the other ways of adding intrinsic attributes to clerical jobs?
4. How should a common or shared philosophy develop in a decentralized, widely spread out organization? If the success of HRD is dependent on the conviction that a manager has about people,

what are the most effective ways of developing these convictions in a dispersed area? What are the strategies likely to be more useful in the Indian context? These questions would need serious experimentation by managers and academicians alike.

5. How should management identify an appropriate entry point for HRD intervention? What are the diagnostic tools for determining the most appropriate strategy for HRD? Singh (1988) has suggested a typology. Further studies in this respect are necessary.

I believe that more organizations are now concerned with HRD than they were a few years ago. I think the difficulty is in translating the concept of HRD into a concrete plan of action. We need in-depth studies and a great deal of experimentation to evolve an appropriate strategy for action

Some useful studies are already being undertaken by HRD Academy at Ahmedabad. Action research in Life Insurance Corporation is reported later in this book. Management Development Institute, Gurgaon has undertaken a study of five organizations which is briefly reported by Sahgal and Jain (1992), and reported in Chapter 1. The study shows that some organizations have integrated HRD philosophy in their management systems, while others have programme-based approach. Survey of HRD practices in Indian organizations are available in many publications (Silvera, 1988; Rao, Verma and Khandelwal, 1988). We would need more evaluative and action research studies.

REFERENCES

Athreya, M.B. (1988). "Integrated HRD Systems-Intervention Strategies" in Rao, T.V. et al. *Alternative Approaches and Strategies of Human Resources Management*. Jaipur: Rawat.

Brown, W. and Jaques, E. (1965). *Glacier Project Papers*. London: Hienemann.

Davis, L.E. and Cherns, A.B. (eds) (1975). *The Quality of Working Life* (Vol. 1), New York: Free Press.

Dayal, I. and Dayal, A.K. (1983). *Organizing for Management*. New Delhi: Concept.

Dayal, I., Srivastava, A. and Alfred, T.M. (1972). *Anatomy of a Strike*. Bombay: Somaiya.

De, N.R. (1984). *Alternative Designs of Human Organizations*. New Delhi: Sage.

McGregor, D. (1966). *Leadership and Motivation*. Cambridge, Mass. MIT Press.

National HRD Network (1989). "Towards Organizational Effectiveness," Conference Papers.

Pigors, P., Myers, C.A. and Malm, F.T. (1959). *Personnel Administration*. New York: McGraw-Hill.

Rice, A.K. (1958). *Productivity and Social Organization: The Ahmedabad Experiment*. London: Tavistock.

Rao, T.V. and Pereira, D.F. (1986). *Recent Experiences in Human Resources Development*, New Delhi: Oxford & IBH.

Rao, T.V., Verma, K.K. Khandelwal, A.K. and Abraham S.J.E. (eds) (1988). *Alternative Approaches and Strategies of Human Resources Management*. Jaipur: Rawat.

Reddin, W.J. (1987). *Effective Management*. New Delhi: Tata McGraw-Hill.

Sahgal, P. and Jain, R. HRD Experiences — Some Case Studies, *MDI Management Journal*, 1992, 5(1): 123-143.

Silvera, D.M. (1988). *Human Resource Development: An Indian Experience*. New Delhi: News India.

Singh, J.P. "Choosing Human Resources Development Interventions", *Vikalpa*, January-March, (1989), 14(1): 35-41.

Strauss, G. and Sayles, L.R. (1985). *Personnel: The Human Problems of Management*. New Delhi: Prentice-Hall.

Trist, E.L. et al. (1963). *Organizational Choice*. London: Tavistock.

4

HRD CLIMATE*

HRD means different things to different organizations. Three things, however, are common to most programmes.

1. Ways to better adjust the individual to his job and the environment;
2. Greater involvement of the employee in various aspects of his work;
3. Greater concern for enhancing the capabilities of the individual.

In essence, HRD approaches have positive values, either explicit or implied,about people and the programmes aim at improving the capabilities of individuals.

Most organizations have begun to recognize that productivity and quality improvement would have to involve people and, in this respect, upgrading the capabilities of employees is essential. Elsewhere, I have discussed (Dayal, 1989) that the expectations of the new entrants from their jobs are different from those of earlier generations. The change is brought about by exposure to the environment, especially the democratic ideas that are propagated through political ideology, the news media, the exposure to TV and other such means. Further, the HRD

* Revised, Original published as ""HRD in Practice: Some Experience and Some Reflections" in *The Indian Journal of Social Work*, Vol LII, No. 4, Oct., 1991. Reproduced by permission.

initiatives are not uniformly successful, and not all organizations have been able to derive or sustain the desired results. Drawing from our research and consulting experience, this chapter identifies some common features of management systems that impede the effectiveness of HRD initiatives. HRD approaches are likely to be sustained in organizations that are able to improve these processes and practices. These are briefly discussed below.

Return-for-Investment Attitude

A number of programmes are started in order to solve certain problems. For example, the Indian Oil Corporation found in their survey that the roles were not clear to its employees. They mounted their HRD initiative around role clarity and role relationships. Crompton Greaves had the need to decentralize their operations and the HRD programme was built around delegation and appraisal. ITC responded to their need for rapid diversification of business by using appraisal as the central point of their HRD programme. In some of these organizations, both the initial efforts and their scope have been enlarged. In some organizations, the scope has remained restricted.

A number of organizations mention that the effectiveness of the HRD programme should be measured in terms of how these efforts contribute to profits. Agarwal (1990) suggests that HRD efforts will be sustained only if the results can improve the profitability of the organization. The Steel Authority of India is actively engaged in developing measures to calculate the contribution made by the HRD programmes in their plants.

Some other organizations take the position that the effectiveness of HRD should be measured in terms of how well the initiatives have contributed to individual growth, and not necessarily to profits. The reason given for the latter is that profits depend upon many factors such as the product, market promotion strategies, technology, managerial decision-making and so on. Higher or lower profits need not necessarily be due to an effective or ineffective HRD system, at least in the short run. Therefore, profits could be high in an organization but HRD may remain ineffective. The link between the two is far from being linear. In fact, for this reason, conceptually, the management has to be clear whether the HRD programme is conditional in the sense that it is supported only if the results show enhanced profits or should the programme effectiveness be measured in terms of human development.

While in most cases HRD has resulted in performance improvement, the measure of effectiveness of the programmes is not always stated in clear terms. In practice many programmes lack conceptual clarity. As a result, appropriate measures of effectiveness of the programme are not developed and relevant data are lacking to evaluate it.

It is, therefore necessary to have an appropriate measure of HRD programme. In its absence it would hardly be possible to know how effective the programme is and what aspects of the programme need improvement. It is indeed true that no programme can be sustained over time if it does not lead to profitability of the enterprise. It should, however, be emphasized that HRD should improve the process of management and the quality of relationships in the organization, which in turn would influence the quality of performance. The appropriateness of the programme will have to be judged in terms of the level of improvement in the management processes and the changes that may have occurred in the quality of interaction among people. Keeping this aspect in view, a number of organizations such as Eicher, Modi Xerox and others carry our annual surveys to judge whether changes in thinking about various aspects of social relationships in the organization have occurred. Profit is an extremely important overall index but insufficient for assessing the effectiveness of specific managerial functions. To measure managerial effectiveness, appropriate indicators have to be developed. The management has to clearly conceptualize the outcome of a particular programme, and develop specific measures to assess its effectiveness.

Concept of Status

In many organizations, status in the managerial hierarchy is near absolute. It is assumed that a person occupying a higher position has superior knowledge and competence in all respects. He feels justified in directing the levels below in what they should or should not do. This pattern of behaviour is maintained even when the subordinate is a specialist. Often, the advice of a specialist is ignored or the superior dictates what the specialists should do. In day-to-day working, the people at various levels have limited freedom of action. Lower levels are not required to exercise discretion. In one organization, officers chosen after a competitive examination were engaged in routine jobs even after 7-8 years of service. They carried out pure routine jobs for their superiors. In essence, the functions of these officers were hardly different from those of the clerical employees. This caused considerable resentment among the officers against the organization and the senior management. In another organization, a specialist was appointed to develop a programme. The management consulted him on certain aspects of the programme but he was never involved in decision-making. He did not even know if his advice was understood fully. In a short while, the specialist began to withdraw from the programme. The examples given here are not exceptional but are common to many organizations. The implicit concept of status and its link to organizational hierarchy does not allow individual growth. The approach interferes with the process of individual development, and therefore the HRD initiatives.

Hierarchy is necessary because different levels of responsibility in organizational tasks is required. The superior and the subordinate each has to have direct responsibility for his level of work. The head of a department would have responsibility for results of that segment of business which falls under his jurisdiction. He will have to assign responsibility for sub-tasks, supervise their performance and provide linkages. The subordinate should be able to exercise full judgement and take decisions in respect to his area of responsibility. The superior should evaluate the quality of discretion used by the subordinate so that the latter can learn from this experience and improve his decision-making capabilities. Each level has a distinct role to perform which is different from other roles in the organization (Jaques, 1962). In many organizations in India the pattern that is most commonly found is that of manger and *assistant to* rather than one of a superior and subordinate manager.

The concept of role boundary is poorly defined in most organizations. This is one of the reasons why persons do not have scope to exercise discretion at lower levels of hierarchy, and have little opportunity to learn from their mistakes. Individual growth is prevented by status-based patterns of behaviour, and styles of functioning at superior and subordinate levels. Such patterns do not generally create or even allow growth-oriented climate in organizations.

Self-orientation

Many managers have the feeling, "We know what is best

for you." The approach "I know best" does not lead to developmental strategies for the employee. Rather an approach like "Why don't you try some other ways" or "Experiment with new approaches" leads to HRD initiatives.

HRD initiatives are unlikely to succeed unless the superior behaves in ways that would facilitate development of the subordinates. The competence and enhanced capabilities of individuals are likely to develop in the context of the work he does. Hence, the quality of diadic relations contribute greatly to the effectiveness of HRD initiatives. Subordinates have to be given freedom to think, to learn from what they do and encouraged to try new ideas. If people are required to do the same job unaltered, they tend to become rooted in routine and are likely to live with a closed mind. HRD programmes cannot be sustained unless operating managers are actively involved in the conduct of the programme. Most successful HRD programmes are spread over the entire organization, and managed by operating managers. The HRD personnel facilitate the process, but rarely manage the programme. The benefits of HRD initiatives should be spread throughout the organization. To do this, each Supervisor would have to assume a developmental approach in dealing with his subordinates. This is the alternative to self-orientation which so commonly interferes with the process of individual development.

Skepticism

The dominant outlook in certain organizations is one of skepticism. Every idea is accompanied with the statement that "we have tried this before, it did not work". This becomes a tradition of certain organizations. Pervasive skepticism develops in an organization for several reasons: the manner in which reports are handled; how problems are solved and how decisions are communicated. Such feelings develop when people suspect that reports are put in cold storage, and programmes started are frequently abandoned. This outlook also develops when people feel that they have no upward influence. In many situations, a skeptical outlook also develops when employees down the line perceive that the management "say one thing and do the opposite".

The most common approach is by appointing a committee to deal with a problem. In many cases committees have limited time to study fully the interconnecting issues, a systemic view. At times the members have a mental set governed by the history of the organization which prevents them from seeking fresh solutions. The reports are examined at the higher levels of management, who accept some recommendations and reject others. At times certain important people do not feel enthusiastic about certain recommendations. In this process the report of the committee is either partially implemented, or ignored completely. When this experience is repeated many times, people in the organization begin to doubt the intentions of the higher management about solving organizational problems. People become skeptical about the management.

Many of the actions of the higher management may be justified. They may be appropriate at the time the decisions are taken. But the reasons are not always understood by the employees where the hierarchy is rigid or no discussion on such matters takes place. In some cases, the management regard such decisions as managerial prerogative and feel that the reasons need not be given to others. Whatever be the logic, people develop skepticism about new initiatives in the organization. HRD initiatives become difficult. Intentions are suspect and people see hidden motives. Some people feel that HRD is one more programme of someone higher up and it would die out in due course.

Culture of Indifference

Some organizations show disregard for schedules, completion of tasks or organizational goals. In meetings, most people seem convinced and agree to take up the programme in right earnest. On return to the desk, the ideas are forgotten unless reminders are sent. The cycle is repeated. In such organizations, committees seldom submit reports on time, nor do individuals. In most situations, no action is taken against the individual or the group for such negligence. The administration shows a state of drift, and individuals at all levels show little concern for achieving organizational goals.

In one organization, the new chief executive who wanted to set new norms of behaviour refused the request of a committee for extension of time. He also asked the committee to make a presentation of a hastily prepared report. The strong criticism of the weaknesses in the proposals made the committee realise what a poor report they had prepared. This incident carried the message in the organization that the committee work and assignments have to be taken more seriously. Along with other changes, the chief executive created awareness among senior employees that they must think about organizational tasks in more purposive ways, and check the drift to which people had become accustomed.

In many organizations, more concern is shown to solve immediate problems and the usual approach is to find expedient solutions. Managers move from one problem to another and in most cases, problems pile up. Managers are so busy seeking immediate solutions that they often lose sight of long-term implications of the solutions. This is more true in administrative areas than in aspects governed by market forces such as product, sales and the like.

In such organizations, HRD takes root slowly. This is so because HRD has a developmental perspective and futuristic orientation. Problem-solving would have to be concerned as much with process as with content so that a more understanding environment is built up within the organization. The manager will have to be concerned with the reasons that may sometimes be covert and not only with the problem as stated. This approach helps the management lay down a foundation for a climate of trust and confidence in relationships among employees.

The managerial processes and practices highlighted here interfere with the goals of HRD initiatives. Effectiveness of HRD is linked with other managerial practices in the organization and cannot be an isolated programme. HRD has to be integrated with the total system.

Rigid Hierarchy Restrict Communication

Open communication is less likely to develop in an organization which has rigid hierarchy and extremely formal patterns of interaction. People lower in the hierarchy would invariably wait for a clue from the superior before expressing an opinion. In one organization, the top management declared that they would like to have an open system, and that officers were welcome to freely approach the members of the higher management. But, in reality, very few people walked through the open doors of the senior officers. Some members of the higher management showed impatience when employees raised questions, and this behaviour conveyed a message contrary to what was said about open communication. Open behaviour develops rarely unless a conductive environment is created for the purpose. In one Union Ministry, the secretariat staff mentioned that when a new Secretary is appointed they wait for his file notings which give them an idea of what he likes, and once the picture is clear, the notes that go to the Secretary are generally in line with what he wants, even if the substance of the new notes is different from those prepared by the same people earlier. This is the way employees adapt to what they perceive as desired or rewarding behaviour. There are organizations which create intense interdepartmental competition. In such organizations, each department develops distinct sub-goals and these lead to interdepartmental conflicts. Group working is rarely possible in such organizations. Competition among departments leads to certain protective attitudes on the part of managers and employees. Given such a situation, cooperation and open relationships receive only a reluctant response.

Some organizations make a sharp distinction between senior officer and clerical categories. These groups would have strong inter-group differences and cooperation among them would be possible only when differences are narrowed down. With the newer generation of employees who are exposed to more egalitarian ideology, such inter-group differences are likely to become sharper. These patterns induce certain kinds of behaviour among employees and these become part of the culture of the organization. These features will have to be recognized and corrective measures taken to develop more cooperative relationships. HRD initiatives will be received with skepticism without any serious attempt to improve the climate of relationships. ITC's example in this aspect is worthy of note. They worked on their organizational problems, communication, etc., along with their HRD initiatives. They followed a well-integrated and overall developmental strategy.

Some organizations pay attention to developing culture that facilitates HRD, while others seem indifferent to the need. In many organizations, certain practices develop in response to certain circumstances at a point of time and these practices later become established. In such cases practices so established often become dysfunctional for developing HRD programmes.

Generally, banks for example, maintain a sharp distinction between Class I and Class III employees. The first group has the responsibility for the transactions that take place; the second group is expected to perform routine operations. A sharp distinction is drawn between the two groups in terms of what is expected of them. This system came into being when banks were small and had limited operations and they also employed less qualified persons in the clerical categories. The picture has now changed. The increased size of banks requires that responsibility be pushed down to lower levels of operatives, clerical employees have nearly the same qualifications as those in Class I. In this kind of situation, HRD would have to deal with inbuilt differences that the organization has created and nurtured.

I have given a few examples of how the social organization in an enterprise develops, and how it facilitates or hinders HRD initiatives. Employees develop patterns of interaction, value systems and organizational norms that are consistent with the organization's culture. Attitudes of employees and how they react to HRD will depend upon the environment of the organization.

Obstacles to HRD Initiatives

The discussion here has highlighted some aspects that hinder HRD initiatives. Many of these features develop when organizations grow in size, or new demands are made upon them by technology or the markets. In many organizations non-competitive, or stable or monopolistic market conditions do not induce conditions for examining internal climate of the organization. There are many organizations, however, that review their systems periodically and make such adjustments as required. Eicher found that their production was stable at a certain level and the efforts to improve the situation met with little success. They invited an outside consultant to help them deal with the situation. They have invited consultants from time to time to look at various problems, and also developed internal capabilities to cope with a variety of new problems. The State Bank of India experienced problems due to rapid expansion and invited a consultant to help them deal with the situation. CMC did not have outside consultants but examined their situation critically and initiated remedial measures as indicated by this examination. With or without a consultant, organizations have to subject themselves to a critical review periodically. Bennis has suggested that organizations have to cultivate a spirit of inquiry, and capability for self-renewal. A number of leading companies in India have carefully studied the new policies of economic liberalization and have prepared plans to cope with the anticipated demands of changing markets and the technology. Tatas, SAIL, Voltas, NOCIL, ITC and many leading companies have carried out exercises to reorient their management systems to cope with future needs of the situation.

Many organizations have found that an exercise on organizational development (OD) is useful prior to, or along with, HRD initiatives. OD is concerned with problems of tasks and relationships in the organization. It has to develop harmony between the demands of the task and the social system, and develop roles and role relationships needed to perform organizational tasks. The OD exercise invariably undertakes diagnosis of the current situation and articulates what new initiatives are required. It takes a comprehensive view of the total system with emphasis on problem solving. In many cases, OD helps in creating the appropriate climate for HRD.

HRD has to be seen from total organizational perspective. Its effectiveness will depend upon how well the programme covers the system as a whole. With years organizations accumulate history and develop traditions. These features of the organization bind them together. These features can also become a handicap to their growth, especially when changes in the wider society are rapid. Organizations have to effectively respond to the demands of the market and bring about changes in the way the work is carried out. If the interpretation of history and tradition is rigid, rather than dynamic, these can become a handicap to growth and not serve as beacon to guide the changes. An organization is likely to remain dynamic if the people are that. This should be the strength of HRD.

REFERENCES

Agarwal, A., "HRD: A Survival Function", *Business India*, July 23 — August 5, 1990.

Dayal, I. "HRD in Indian Organisations: Current Perspectives and Future Issues", *Vikalpa*, 14(4), 1989.

Dayal, I., "Role Analysis Technique in Job Descriptions", *California Management Review*, XI, (4), 1969.

Jaques, E. (1961). Equitable Payment. London, Heinemann.

Miller, E.J. and Rice, A.K. (1967). *Systems of Organisation*. London: Tavistock.

Schein, E.H. (1985). *Organisational Culture and Leadership*. San Francisco: Jossey-Bass.

5

DESIGNING HRD INTERVENTIONS*

1

The HRD system has roots in the concepts of quality of work life and quality circles, not just welfare-oriented ideology. It emphasizes psychological growth of the individual besides security and physical well-being. The concept of psychological growth has to do with enhancement of the individual's capacity to deal with his situation. It improves his competence, skills, enhances his maturity and adjustment to the environment. The programme should give him confidence and develop his capacity to adjust well to a rapidly changing situation.

While HRD is based on humanistic beliefs (Dayal, 1989), the need for it is increasingly felt by organizations on account of two emerging realities: one, the need to effectively respond to the changing nature of expectations of people joining the labour force. Younger employees seem to need more independence, develop their own identity and require a clearer definition of rights rather than dependence on their employers for their well-being. They need more elbow room to express themselves. The welfare and paternal approaches satisfy the younger generations entering the job market less than they did the earlier generations. This is due to changes in society and in child-rearing practices, at least in urban and semi-urban environment. The habit of self-appraisal and

---

1. * Based on an article Dayal, I., "Designing an HRD Programme" in *Excellence Through Human Resource Development*, M.R.R. Nair and T.V. Rao, (Ed.), Tata Mcgraw-Hill, New Delhi, 1990, pp. 116-125.

confidence in one's own abilities develops from early childhood experiences. These characteristics will sharpen as child-rearing practices change. With changes in aspirations, employees would have to simultaneously develop a sense of responsibility for, and involvement in organizational goals. The managerial and supervisory practices would have to induce this sense of involvement or what has been called a spontaneous will to cooperate. Organizations will have to respond constructively to the changing aspirations of employees.

Besides the changing nature of employee expectations, the second consideration is that organizational survival would require increasingly higher capacity to adjust to change and newness. The process of adjustment would be smoother in organizations that have movement, promote a spirit of inquiry and have an atmosphere of learning. HRD is a managerial response to the corporate need. This explains why technology-based and growth organizations have paid more attention to HRD than others (Silvera, 1988).

The HRD perspective would have to consist of more than humanistic or welfare direction. The psychological growth would require involvement of the individual in the process of learning. An HRD programme that centres around growth of a person as a total being has to keep in view several factors. This chapter discusses some basic considerations necessary in the designing and operating an HRD programme. Five design considerations are discussed in this chapter. They are:

(1) Learning Process
(2) Cultural Factor
(3) Managerial Orientation
(4) Administrative Strategy
(5) Supervision

1. Learning Process

The factors that contribute to learning have to be considered in the design and operation of an HRD programme.

(i) *Relational Factors*

An individual does not learn in isolation. He learns from interaction with others. Hence the quality and variety of interaction are important for learning. Chris Argyris (1964) has emphasized that an individual learns about himself by the way other people react to him. In this sense other people are a mirror to him for understanding himself. In some cases other people serve as a role model. More open the interaction among people, higher the probability that an individual will learn about himself from such interactions. This is one important reason why HRD programmes pay special attention to diadic and group experiences. The programme must influence the climate of interaction among employees at all three levels, the diadic, the group and the organization as a whole. In a number of organizations these aspects become a part of separate programmes such as counselling, improvement in internal communication, group and intergroup problem-solving meetings, etc. Results of these efforts contribute significantly to the success of HRD initiatives in an organization. In this sense such efforts become an integral part of HRD. Experiences at all these levels contribute significantly to an individual's growth. Each level is complementary to the other levels. At times a preoccupation with group processes tends to ignore the significant role that individuals play in an organization (Dayal, 1970). Total attention of the individual without equal attention to a group also hinders relationships that are necessary for self-development. Attention to both individual and group processes is important for organizational health.

(ii) *Experience for Learning*

Self-confidence, competence and skill develop from doing things oneself and not by thinking about what can be done. A theorem appears clear enough when a student reads a chapter in a mathematics book, but he is unlikely to be able to use it effectively unless he solves the practical examples at the end of the chapter. Laboratory work is necessary to learn the concepts in physics, engineering, medical sciences and many other applied areas of study. Management schools are using business games, projects and a variety of experience-based teaching methods to provide relevant experience to students and enhance his learning. In administration likewise experience of doing the job is necessary to gain confidence. Experience of confronting problems in handling a variety of situations is an important input for maturation. A person who has not handled problems and issues tends to oversimplify them. Often a person changes his perspective when he is placed in a position to handle problems himself. Many times a manager finds that things that looked obvious and simple from a distance are in fact not so. Decision-making and problem-solving are requirements for maturation and self-learning. HRD programmes would have, therefore, to provide a variety of meaningful experiences to employees to develop competence and skill to handle effectively work-related problems.

Experience is also important for an individual to learn values, attitudes, meaning of work, norms of behaviour and the like. An individual learns the right and wrong standards of behaviour through interactions with peers, superiors and subordinates, and from what he observes in his environment of work (Argyris, 1964, 1957). This is the process of organizational socialization. As new-comers learn the norms of behaviour, attitudes and values from their interactions with other people, certain patterns of behaviour are perpetuated from one generation of employees to another. These patterns constitute the culture of the organization.

If values and attitudes have to change, as in an organization development (OD) programme, the patterns of interaction in the organization would have to change. This is why OD programmes emphasize simultaneous changes in the structure of work, control and supervisory practices, distribution of power and authority and definition of responsibility at work. These changes induce new patterns of interaction and, in turn, bring about changes in attitudes and values and in the perspectives about work. HRD has to provide new experiences, new patterns of interaction for inducing new learning.

Two considerations for growth and development seem necessary:

(a) An individual must be involved personally in the process of development and know what new learning could lead to his growth.
(b) The organization would have to provide a variety of experiences to an individual to learn from these experiences.

(iii) *Need to Learn*

The third aspect of learning process is that an individual should have motivation to grow. He should sharpen his capacity to learn and have the urge to improve his individual effectiveness. In many organizations, individuals perform routine and repetitive tasks. The jobs have ill-defined boundaries with the result that the subordinate functions mainly as an *assistant to* the manager and constantly checks whether he can take one or the other decision. The boundaries of several roles overlap. There is no discreteness between one level of job and another. Given such conditions, individuals develop a mechanical view of the job. In our interviews, managers have referred to these as jobs which require no thinking, or initiative. The mind is set into a mould and most decisions are taken within the parameters determined by precedence and rules. In such organizations the decisions are taken at high levels and individuals develop an unthinking standard approach to work. Desire for personal growth, acquisition of new knowledge, self-confidence and such patterns are less likely to develop in an environment that have these features. Desire to learn has a great deal to do with the environment at work. If routinization of a job takes away initiative and discretion from the job, a programme like HRD alone can hardly develop an urge to grow. Roles and role boundary would have to be studied and rationalized. It would be necessary to examine jobs to avoid what Reddin (1987) has called one-over-one task responsibility, i.e., a superior repeats a great deal of what the subordinate does. In this situation the subordinate is unlikely to feel the responsibility for results because the review of his work takes place within a short span of time by his superior (Jaques, 1961). It is observed that generally jobs become mechanical and people lack initiative in organizations where work is organized on one-over-one basis. Initiative develops when the person is required to exercise judgement in performing his job. This concept is now extensively used in designing work systems in Japan and the most successful companies in the West.

2. **Cultural Factor**

Generally Indian child-rearing practices induce

dependence. Children have limited scope for appraising their strengths and limitations and developing self-reliance. The patterns of interaction in schools, social institutions and colleges reinforce dependence on people in positions of authority (Chattopadhyay, 1975; Sinha, 1988; Dayal, 1976). These patterns are slowly changing and they would perhaps be different in the next 20/25 years. In the social environment of many Indian organizations, the concept of growth assumes two forms: (i) by presenting a role model, the superior officer expects his subordinate to become like himself, and (ii) by constant inducement and direction the superior officer moulds the subordinate to become an ideal person, as per his model. HRD has a different concept of growth. This concept hypothesizes that the dynamics of growth of individuals is different. A person would grow best if he is to find his own mould. One person may learn from taking up an impossible challenge; another person will learn from incremental effort. An individual should understand his own strengths and weaknesses, and analyse the reasons for both. He should evolve a personal strategy to improve his own capability. This approach is referred to here as clinical approach.

The directional approach makes heavy demands on the supervisor as he would have to either be a role model or take up responsibility for directing an individual's growth. He will have to constantly monitor the behaviour of the individual. In this model responsibility for growth shifts from the individual to the supervisor.

In the clinical approach, the superior takes up the responsibility to create conditions at work that enable the individuals to grow. He is concerned with influencing those elements of the management that facilitate self-development for employees. These elements consist of the climate of learning, job design so that an individual can learn from his experience, a positive climate for interaction, personnel practices that serve the needs of employees, and the like. HRD programmes have this orientation.

3. **Managerial Orientation**

A number of managers believe that the mission of an enterprise is producing goods and services at a profit. People are seen to be a means to achieving the results. Those employees who contribute to the production of goods and services deserve the manager's attention. Poor producers could be ignored. This is a selective approach. The consequences of a selective approach are many and are extensively discussed in the literature (Sherif, 1967). Differentiation contributes to factionalism among employees, hostility among factions, poor communication and undesired forms of competition. It leads to *we* and *they* feeling making homogeneous social organization difficult. The inter-group conflict and hostility create mistrust and due to this, cooperation among them is difficult to establish.

HRD does not follow selective approach. Rather it has belief in developing all people to their full capacity. The programmes that enable growth are meant for all employees. It is true that some employees will invest less in their growth than others and, therefore, benefit from the programme in proportion to what they put into it. But this option is exercised by the individual and not the organization.

4. **Administrative Strategy**

The effectiveness of HRD depends on implementation. There would have to be goal-sharing among managers. In some organizations goal-sharing in HRD has to be consciously developed. The implementation strategy would have to help them examine their belief about people and work. It would have to transform the thinking.

Impressions often grow into convictions about work and people from what colleagues say about these, and from personal experiences in handling day-to-day problems. The manager has to cope with many irritants at work: indiscipline, low efficiency or quality, lack of concern for maintaining schedules, need to coax people to finish their assigned jobs and many other stresses occasioned by work flow and work related problems. The manager's beliefs are based on how he interprets his experiences, and how he responds to events that he observes. In training situations, change in thinking comes about by rearranging experiences and data and interpreting these in new ways. From this exercise new insights develop. This process requires discussions and an opportunity to re-evaluate one's own beliefs and values. The exercise needs time, patience and perseverance. The strategy to implement the HRD approach would have to initiate a process of *thinking and self-appraisal.*

Most organizations have found that changes in one's perception about work and people are triggered through changes in the way controls are exercised, and in the decision-making and problem-solving practices (Simon, 1945; Tannenbaum, 1962). When the superior officer controls performance both in terms of what is achieved (content) and how (process), the subordinate becomes more aware of what kind of interactions he ought to notice, and perhaps initiate. In problem-solving as well, remedial measures are employed not only for the apparent but also for the motivating reasons for an event or behaviour. Problem-solving strategies have to deal with the cause and *not* the symptom. In decision-making also, alternatives have to be examined and the choice is made with awareness of its short- and long-term consequences. When senior managers emphasize these aspects in their dealings with subordinates, a chain reaction is set in and the subordinate is encouraged to think through problems, and reappraise his experiences. Many organizations have initiated short programmes for managers to develop a common framework for analysing work-related and human problems.

5. **Supervision**

A great deal has been written on supervisory leadership. A supervisor is man-in-the-middle. He is generally on the receiving end. Where trade unions are strong, the middle and junior levels of officers in managerial positions experience intense stress. A large number of managers feel that in the absence of authority to freely reward and punish employees, they cannot get work from them. In essence many managers feel that subordinates should implicitly follow the wishes of their superiors, and anyone who questions these is to be seen as a "difficult" employee. In interviews and discussions managers say that the subordinate should be afraid of or be in awe of his superior and in the absence of this it is not possible to get him to work. This is a widely shared view. Consistent with this belief, the superiors concept of *control* is regulating behaviour of the subordinate, not results.

This view is formed due to a number of reasons:

(i) Authority and power are equated in most Indian organizations. Authority is in fact an attribute of the position, while power is an attribute of the individual. If a person can influence another person to do what he wants him to do, he has power over him. In a well-functioning bureaucracy, authority and power are equated. In most organizations this hypothetical position does not prevail. Because a manager's position has authority built into the position, he assumes that he could also automatically influence the subordinate's behaviour. He could of course have coercive power, i.e. to selectively reward or punish a person, and by virtue of this, influence his behaviour. In modern organizations, however, the coercive power that the management had and employed at work, has led to counter-coercive forces such as trade unions, civil rights legislation, constitutional protection, etc. In modern society coercive power is generally resented and often censored.

A manager has to behave and function in ways that gains him influence over his subordinates. The influence, in a manner of speaking, has to be earned; it is not inherent in a manager's position. He has to earn the confidence of the subordinates by giving each one pride in himself as a person.

(ii) Discriminatory practices between different groups of people gives rise to *we* and *they* feelings. These practices create alienation between the manager and the employees he supervises. In this kind of situation, suspicion and distrust rather than mutual confidence and trust develop. With this development, both the supervisor and the supervised feel the need for coercive power.

(iii) The feeling that fear and distance are needed to control people is often an outcome of managerial styles and that of the assumptions managers have about people. Many organizations are beginning to explore their assumptions about people and develop practices that are consistent with these beliefs. CMC, for example, believes that each person should be responsible for his own performance. The supervisor should equip the subordinate with training, and provide him with services that would enable him to do his job well, and allow him sufficient autonomy to achieve expected results. Eicher has developed participative practices where responsibility at work is shared. They emphasize the need for group working, and recognition of interdependence as against individual orientation. Transformational leadership studies (Singh and Bhandarkar, 1990) show that the leader's significant contribution has been in removing obstructions from the subordinate's environment, and setting high goals of achievement. These experiences are repeated in many organizations such as BHEL, Nyveli Lignite Corporation, Steel Authority of India and others.

Developing participative systems needs a great deal of faith and patience. The participants show many trends that tend to discourage efforts to develop these practices in many organizations. Some of the discouraging factors are:

(i) The participants have pat answers to problems without carefully examining data. The habit of using data and systematically analysing situations comes slowly, and patience is needed to develop these habits.

(ii) Most people who have not handled independent responsibility, often indulge in sweeping generalizations and assume a "we know better" attitude. In time with persistent effort this attitude mellows down. Participative systems develop through a process of maturation.

(iii) The transition from a distant observer to an active participant is often made difficult due to affiliations to, or influence of, one's representative group. Objectivity in discussions has to be consciously developed.

The development of participative systems needs planning and preparation. Sinha's (1988) research shows that organizations which have developed participative practices in stages have succeeded better than those who have moved straightaway to participative structures. In Stage I a more permissive, guided, training-oriented development may lead to Stage II where full-scale participation is encouraged. Jaques (1951) reports that intensive developmental efforts were needed at Glacier to make participative systems effective.

HRD is both a philosophy and a vision and a guide to managerial action. It is not a technique but a comprehensive programme to translate the philosophy into practice. It deals with the minds of men, and covers the organization as a whole. The much praised Japanese work systems are consistent with the ideas discussed in this chapter. The worker is given responsibility for results. He is, for example, responsible for many of the operations that contribute to results, such as machine setting, routine maintenance, quality measurement and the like. He is involved in various aspects of the work through quality circle. His involvement is persuaded through work practices, and not by separate programmes. An employee is required to exercise his judgement and think about his job.

The design of HRD interventions would have to comprehend certain important considerations such as the following:

1. HRD is not a technique. It is based on management's beliefs about people. The translation of the idea may require specific programmes, and use of certain established techniques that may contribute to the realization of the goals of HRD.
2. HRD interventions would require attention to several aspects of work organization such as

design of jobs, communication, supervisory practices, etc. and not personnel practices alone.

3. Responsibility for growth is that of the individual but the management has to create conditions for growth. In facilitating growth, process interventions are more effective than direct control.
4. HRD must involve the total organization and not segments of the population.
5. HRD can achieve its goals when the operating managers share the belief and assume responsibility for results. It is not a specialist function except in terms of designing, initiating, promoting and evaluating the programme.

REFERENCES

Argyris Chris (1964). *Integrating the Individual and the Organisation*, Willey, New York.

Argyris Chris (1957). *Personality and Organisation*, Harper, New York.

Chattopadhyay, C.P. "Dependency in Indian Culture from Mud Huts to Company Board Rooms", *Econ. & Pol. Weekly*, 1975, 19(22).

Dayal, I. "Some Dilemmas in Newer Concepts of Administration", *California Management Review*, 1970, 13(1).

Dayal, I. (1976). *Change in Work Organisation*, Concept, New Delhi.

Jaques, E. (1961). *Equitable Payment*, Heinemann, London.

Jaques, E. (1951). *Changing Culture of Factory*, Tavistock, London.

Reddin, W.J. (1987). *Effective Management*, Tata McGraw-Hill, New Delhi.

Sheriff, M. (1967). *Group Conflict and Co-operation*, Routledge & Kegal Paul, London.

Silvera, D.M. (1988). *Human Resource Development: The Indian Experience*, New India Publications, New Delhi.

Simon, H.A. (1945). *Administrative Behaviour*, Macmillan, London.

Singh P. & Bhandarkar, A. (1990). *Corporate Success and Transformational Leadership*, Wiley Eastern, New Delhi.

Sinha, J.B.P. (1988). *Work Culture in Indian Organisation*, A.N. Sinha Institute of Social Studies, Patna (Mimeograph).

Tannenbaum, A. "Control of Organisations: Individual Adjustment and Organisational Performance", *Admin. Science Qtly*, 1962, 7(2): 236-257.

6

HRD IN LIC

Experience of the Life Insurance Corporation (LIC) illustrates some of the ideas discussed in earlier chapters. I shall first briefly discuss the background of the Corporation and the history of earlier efforts to improve the system before detailing the main features of their HRD Programmes.

LIC has a four-tier organization. The central office, which is located in Bombay, seven zonal offices, about 92 divisional offices and nearly 2000 branches. It employs about 100,000 employees, of which 10,000 are Class I officers. The Corporation was created in 1956 by an Act of Parliament. Under the Act the life insurance business was nationalized. Hence, LIC merged all the companies that were carrying on life business.

In the 70s the growth of business was slow. The Corporation had been subjected to strong public criticism. There were several internal and external committees to look into the affairs and many changes were made without appreciable improvement in its performance. The Chairman of LIC in 1978, Mr. J. Matthan, writes, "By early seventies, there was a deep malaise affecting the Life Insurance Corporation of India. The enthusiasm of the early days had all but vanished. The Corporation, which was described in mid-sixties, by Shri Jawaharlal Nehru as the success story of the public sector, was just limping along". And later, "When T.A. Pai became Chairman, an attempt was made at restructuring the organization through implementing the recommendations of an internal committee—the Nayudu Committee—but this attempt proved abortive, mainly because many in senior management were not convinced about the wisdom and practicability of the restructuring proposals. By the time I took over as Chairman in 1978, it was obvious to all in top management that morale was at low ebb and that something needed to be done urgently to improve performance" (R.K. Talwar, *Tributes*, p. 54).

In mid-1980s the author was invited as consultant to help LIC work on its problems and this led to major reorganization of the Corporation (Balachandran, 1987). While it is not the purpose here to examine the details of organizational development efforts at LIC, the special features of this reorganization that have a direct bearing on the strategy employed later for HRD initiatives will be useful to summarize.

1. The distinct features of the new organization were:

   (i) The four-tier organization consisting of the central, zonal, divisional and branch offices was considered necessary. However, the purpose of each office was redefined. These were classified as follows:

Office	Purpose
Central Office	Policy formulation and corporate planning and review.
Zonal Office	Headquarters office for all operating matters and development of inputs needed for ensuring future growth.
Divisional Office	Control of and service to branch offices.
Branch Office	Operating office with responsibility for profit and growth.

(ii) The branches were responsible for profit and growth from being primarily a sales outlet earlier. The change of definition entailed total reorganization and reorientation of the branch offices. All functions that significantly contribute towards profit and customer service were shifted to the branch. Branch became the single point of contact for the customer. The sales, new business underwriting, policy-holder servicing, accounting and office services including machine records were shifted from divisional to branch offices. The size of the two offices also changed. The divisional offices became smaller and branch offices larger.

(iii) A system of performance budget and review was introduced to exercise controls through results and provide a greater measure of autonomy at operating levels.

(iv) The divisional offices were reorganized to provide technical service, advice and exercise effective control over branch performance.

(v) Plans for reorganizing central and zonal offices were prepared but for special reasons they could not be implemented until later.

(vi) The reorganization was designed to

(a) Strengthen the middle levels of management in both branch and devisional offices. Each department was to be small enough for the departmental head concerned to develop close relationships with employees in the department and provide effective supervision.

(b) Define and write down roles in each office. In devising the roles, care was taken to avoid one-over-one position, i.e. two persons in hierarchical positions handling the same work. Each role would have responsibility for results as defined in the Role Analysis. This arrangement would give responsibility for results at each level of the hierarchy.

(c) Clarify the linkages and interdependence between roles. The Role Analysis consisted of three parts: the first part defined the purpose of the role—what should the particular role contribute to the totality; the second part identified the prescribed elements; the third part laid down the areas of discretion needed to serve the purpose for which the position was created (Dayal, 1969).

(vii) Keeping in view the size of LIC, the reorganization plans were implemented in three phases. In Phase I, the experimental phase, three divisions were take up followed by 21 divisions in Phase II and the remaining divisions in Phase III. A cell at the central office to help the top management and small cells of 2/3 officers in each division were created to facilitate implementation. LIC also mounted special training programmes for its officers who were involved in the proposed changes.

The Emerging Situation

The reorganization helped LIC to accelerate its growth from around 12 per cent to 35 per cent and substantially expand the business. With rapid growth the Corporation had to seriously examine how to manage growth.

Managing Growth

The management of LIC had to initiate action to deal with the problems of growth. Several steps were taken to further decentralize operations and enhance financial powers at lower levels. Apart from setting up additional branch, divisional and zonal offices, and increasing the field force and all other categories of employees, the management decided that greater attention to development of people in the corporation was required. This was necessary because (i) improvement in the quality of service would depend on the involvement of the employee in his job, and this in turn would depend on how he feels about the work he does and his sharing, at least in general terms, the goals of the corporation, and (ii) Integration of new employees with the older ones had to be smooth and both groups should feel that they are valued by the management.

There was need to think constructively about human resources in the Corporation. A systematic examination of this question began with the formulation of LIC's Personnel Policy. Two steps were taken:

1. After Extensive discussions at different levels, a document to lay down the personnel policy was prepared. The policy also articulated the management's beliefs about people.
2. A survey of training needs was undertaken. A sample of 2000 drawn from all levels of employees in different locations was undertaken. Based on the findings of this survey, a document on LIC's Training Policy was prepared. To implement the policy, the strength of the Officers Training Centre in Bombay was doubled and six Zonal Training Centres were created in each of the six zonal headquarters. About 21 Sales Training Centres were also set up for training of field personnel. Special attention was paid to developing training material, improving quality of instruction and placement of instructors.

A Task Force worked on the strategy to implement the Personnel Policy. Seven programmes were identified to realize the goals of the Personnel Policy. Task forces were created at the central and zonal offices to implement the programmes. The seven programmes were:

1. Developing and testing Manpower Forecasting Model.
2. Review of personnel practices to bring them in line with the goals stated in the Personnel Policy.
3. Human Resource Development.
4. Training at all levels.
5. Review industrial relations and develop collaborative practices with trade unions.
6. Improving internal communication.
7. Redesign jobs at all levels.

Task groups were organized in interlocking teams as the tasks were interdependent. While developing each programme, there was also need to keep the linkages in perspective.

HRD Interventions

The policy articulated the beliefs about people (Policy Statement in LIC) as follows:

"(i) Development of a person and an employee at work cannot be segmented into separate categories. HRD has to be concerned with a person as a total being. HRD should have to be concerned with developing the ability of the individual and his adjustment to the total environment.

(ii) Experience is the most important way of learning new ways, hence development would have to provide new and varied experiences to the individual.

(iii) HRD is a philosophy of life in the organization and must be reflected in all aspects of management. Since LIC is a large organization, it would be necessary to have a distinct programme or a series of programmes that would help the organization achieve the goal of human development.

(iv) HRD programme should be developed keeping these considerations in view."

The group on HRD sub-tasks examined the practical implications of these beliefs and decided after considerable discussion that the characteristics of the programmes should be the following:

> HRD should provide growth experience to individuals. The meaning of growth for this programme is comprehensive. It includes development of an individual's strengths, enhanced capability to adjust to his environment, acquiring new skills and a broader perspective of work and society. Growth does not mean only promotion in the job, though promotion is to be seen as recognition of his capabilities as compared to others in his group. Growth is a more comprehensive idea than just promotion on the job.
>
> The growth may be experienced by a variety of inputs such as new assignments, training, involvement in improving his method of doing work, enhanced skills through interaction with others, and so on. The learning is likely to take place when certain conditions are provided: a manager thinks about what is done well by him and what is done poorly, articulates his strengths and weaknesses, takes steps to overcome his weaknesses and strengthen further

his strengths, and reviews how useful his efforts have been. This is the process that would create a learning situation for the manager and the organization should create conditions to operationalize this process. The learning experience has to be preferably built into the job itself, because that is the most significant concern of an employee at work. The nature of this involvement should be such as to facilitate self-development.

The HRD interventions mainly consisted of the following:

(i) Strengthening internal communication through written, visual and face-to-face media. The central and zonal offices started newsletters, a video-news programme and small group meetings.

(ii) *Review of Appraisal System*: The present system should be reviewed to make the appraisee a party to the review of his performance. The exercise of developing the new system must involve the representatives of the officers.

(iii) *Career Planning*: A detailed programme for career planning is necessary where the individual concerned should be involved in exercising his career choice.

(iv) *Succession Planning*: Carefully planning succession for about 200 senior and top-level positions and give them well-planned experience and training for positions of higher responsibility. These positions will include specialist jobs as well.

(v) *Job Redesign*: Undertaking redesign of jobs in the central and zonal offices to provide a greater degree of autonomy and direct responsibility for results. These positions should be concerned with corporate- level policy, review, future development, systems improvement, manpower development and such other activities as would ensure continuing growth of LIC.

The job redesign will have to be undertaken at the divisional and branch levels later.

(vi) Systematic plans of training all levels of employees and agents as per the Training Policy.

(vii) Counselling training to senior and middle level managers with the objective of influencing the climate of interaction at diadic and group levels.

(viii) Suggestion scheme to encourage innovative ideas.

(ix) *Work Planning and Review System (W.P.-R.)*: This system was developed to involve an individual think about his job, appraise it and plan what he needs to do to improve overall performance in relation to his own role. It has five components, as follows:

(i) Surveying the job to identify strengths and weaknesses in performance. A departmental head in a Divisional Office, for example, would have to survey the strengths and weakness in branches under the Division in his functional area, and determine how these weak branches can overcome their shortcomings.

(ii) Planning action in concrete terms to help the weaker branches improve their technical and administrative capabilities in short- and long-term context, and his specific contribution in this direction.

(iii) Developing a measure of effectiveness or otherwise of his interventions.

(iv) After planning his work, a discussion with his supervisor and six-monthly review of performance by himself and later with the supervisor.

(v) Identification of areas where the individual would want to develop certain skills and capabilities, and the help needed from the superior officer in this respect.

The W.P.-R. was an important instrument of self-development. It was developed after considerable discussion and experimentation. The logic underlying this programme may be useful for understanding how it was seen as an instrument of self-development. It assumed that growth experience should be linked to the central activity in which people are involved. This activity relates to the organizational roles that managers perform. The individual should conceptualize what he wants to achieve, plan how he is going to do it, and measure how well he has succeeded. This process of thinking and evaluating in concrete terms would enhance the analytical and evaluative capabilities of the individual. The exercise will also show up what new areas of knowledge, skills, capabilities he wants to develop, and seek help from his superior officer to acquire them.

The earlier exercise by LIC to reorganize roles was effectively used to develop W.P.-R. system. The consideration could be summarized in the following way:

> Each job has a purpose for which it is created. This purpose defines the boundary of the job, called Role Boundary. As the purpose of one job is different from other jobs, the Role Boundary of each job is distinct. The role incumbent is given freedom to exercise his discretion within his role boundary to achieve results. And in doing so, the individual can be relatively autonomous, innovative and resourceful. The quality of discretion would determine the quality of results that the individual would achieve. Further, discussion of results with a sympathetic superior will provide the

subbordinate greater understanding of his own strengths and weaknesses, and improve his capacity for self-appraisal. The individual plans for results within his role boundary and reviews his achievements and failures with his superior officer. The W.P.-R. is used as an instrument for self-development, and not for performance appraisal.

The initiative for self-development through W.P.-R. is the individual's. The management has created an environment for this purpose by redesigning jobs, defining role-boundary and providing autonomy to the individual to exercise discretion within the role boundary. The total exercise involves the operating managers, though training in skills needed to review W.P.-R., in counselling and other related areas is arranged by the HRD Task Force.

Implementation

While other sub-systems such as appraisal, career planning, etc. were being developed and discussed with representative bodies, wherever required, the initiatives began with W.P.-R. The concept of W.P.-R. came out of the characteristics that the Task Group had laid down in earlier discussions. The ideas had to be operationalized and made an integral part of the day-to-day work of the manager. The Group worked on a system that would help a manager to *think* about his job, identify what needs to be done to improve the situation and devise ways of doing this. This thinking led to the idea of Work Planning and Review System. The key responsibility for undertaking this exercise rested with the individual. The Group decided to develop a format and try out the system in one of the seven zonal offices and cover only the senior people in the first phase.

The proposal was presented to and discussed by the

top management. The programme was to cover about 100 senior managers in one of the seven Zonal offices. The purpose of the try-out was to test the underlying assumption of the programme, method of implementation and its effectiveness. These aspects of the programme would be studied in-depth before extending it to other offices. This approach was found useful as many important changes in the programme were made, which improved its quality.

The implementation strategy included the following:

1. Discussion of the proposal in a two-day Seminar for members of the representative organization of officers.
2. Preparation of audio-visual material for use in the Seminar.
3. Three two-day Seminars to cover all 100 managers to discuss the rationale of W.P.-R. and the operating details.
4. Setting up a Task Force in the Central office and Zonal office to conduct the Seminars, and the follow up. The responsibility for implementation will rest with the in-charge of the Zone; the members of the Task Force will help in carrying out specified tasks.
5. Detailed study of the implementation to be undertaken after three months and at regular intervals after that.
6. Programme of intensive training for members of the Task Force.
7. Regular feed-back to be provided to the top management.

Two-day seminars were arranged with the help of an outside consultant, starting with senior managers. This exercise had two purposes: (i) to train senior persons first so that they know what W.P.-R. aims to do, and what is expected of them, and (ii) package a programme for use of the members of the Task Force who would be conducting these seminars throughout the Corporation.

It was decided that implementation of major programmes is best done in face-to-face meetings. It is necessary for people to know the rationale of the proposals, discuss the programme and have an opportunity to discuss it with colleagues. The capsule had a number of group and role play exercises for people to examine their doubts and apprehensions about the programme.

The Career Planning, the W.P.-R., and the appraisal system were at present designed for managerial jobs. For categories engaged on clerical jobs, the communication, suggestion scheme, training, counselling and job design were considered more useful. The job design had to be coordinated with the trade unions.

HRD is located in thc Personnel Department of LIC. It is a separate division, as are Personnel, Industrial Relations and Manpower Planning. It provides specialist inputs only, as the real responsibility for HRD rests with the operating managers. The essential features of the implementation strategy were the following:

1. Extensive consultation in devising the main elements of the HRD programme.
2. Experimenting in smaller units the programmes such as W.P.-R. and other sub-systems of HRD before full-scale implementation, and improving the quality of the programme from this experience.
3. Training members of a Task Force who would carry out face-to-face discussion with officers on HRD instruments. A Task Force is created in each zonal office and in the central office.
4. Monitoring the programme in all locations of the

Corporation.

5. Conducting special programmes, called ownership workshops, for the Divisional Managers, Marketing Managers and others so that they can take over the responsibility to effectively operate the HRD programme, and ensure agreed results.
6. Undertaking studies from time to time to assess the effectiveness of the HRD programme.
7. When the programmes are fully operationalized, disband the Task Force.

Difficulties in Implementation

The experience in LIC suggests that the management has to constantly monitor and deal with two kinds of realities. Many of the points mentioned below were highlighted in research and in review meetings, and appropriate corrective measures taken by the management.

Managerial Issues

(i) There is a tendency to ignore role boundary of one's own and that of other roles, especially in superior-subordinate situations. Not many superiors have the perspective and self-confidence to facilitate a subordinate's learning by allowing him to exercise discretion and learn from his own mistakes. Instead the superior gives detailed instructionas and wants the job done as he would have done himself. LIC experience shows that in situations where the appropriate style of supervision and respect for role autonomy have not developed, the concept of growth through W.P.-R. has not significantly occurred. This aspect has to receive constant attention by the higher management and the Task Force.

(ii) Short-term perspectives in handling day-to-day problems create new problems, and over time, they tend to pile up. In many cases more rules are made to deal with new situations and, over time, a plethora of rules overtake discretion, making a job routine and repetitive. Many steps have been taken to develop long-term perspectives in problem solving and this aspect has to be reviewed frequently by the top management and the Task Force.

(iii) While jobs have a discretionary element built into them, at times in day-to-day working discretion is not fully respected by supervisors. In this way jobs become highly mechanical. Care has to be taken that role boundaries are reviewed whenever new tasks are created. It is often found that an office which tends to minimize managerial discretion also routinizes functions and shows low innovativeness in performance. Such units also tend to have an "inner" orientation, more concern for the procedure than the market or external situation. All these aspects of management tend to become counter-productive for HRD. It is difficult to graft practices that promote individual growth in this kind of environment. Hence, freeing up the organization from rigidity is necessary to have effective HRD interventions. LIC's Task Force has a clear mandate to identify these processes and take remedial measures where necessary. These efforts have succeeded in some cases but not always. The Task Force carries out independent research studies to evaluate the situation and provide feedback to top management for decisions on new strategies that might become necessary.

(iv) Appropriate supervisory practices are most important in the HRD programme. Intensive programmes of training have helped some but developmental aspects of the managerial role in many cases is a long way from developing. In cases where this awareness has developed, HRD initiatives have been more effective.

Personal Issues

(i) Some managers are used to being told what to do and find it difficult to take up direct responsibility, and accept autonomy. The individual counselling programme has to cope with this problem. Small group meetings by the Task Force also has to deal with this problem.

(ii) It is difficult for some people to think in terms of results. People are more comfortable reacting to situations as they come. Planning for results requires that the manager concerned must establish collaborating relations with those who precede or succeed the operations. These are work flow relationships. He has to think in terms of networking with other managers. This also requires interpersonal and negotiating skills. Attention to these aspects has to be often drawn by the Task Force. This aspect is emphasized in the W.P.-R. system and is spreading slowly, and needs constant review by the Task Force.

Lessons

The experience of LIC suggests that HRD cannot be regarded as an isolated programme. It must become a way of life in the Corporation. It must involve all parts and cover all people in the organization. In LIC, HRD followed the organizational development programme. This sequence helped in several ways, namely,

(i) it created an environment to extensively question the meaning of human development;
(ii) having defined roles and role boundary earlier, the W.P.-R. system could be evolved in its present form;
(iii) the success of the organizational development efforts created conditions for acceptance of HRD

and willingness to experiment with new ideas.

Experimentation with ideas was accepted as a normal approach for such programmes. Due to this approach, many significant changes were brought about in the programme, making it more suitable for the situation.

The review and monitoring system developed by LIC was very useful. The Task Force has played a crucial role in the development and implementation of the programme. The research studies and review by top and senior management have played an important role in the entire HRD programme. The research studies are carried out by the Task Force and discussed by top management. In the annual top management Seminar, the findings of research are presented, and discussed at length. The discussion leads to a plan of action to strengthen or enlarge the scope of the programme. The role of the members of the Seminar is also discussed, and the help that they should give is clearly identified. At times independent assessment of the programme is made by the consultant and the findings are discussed. Review of the programme is also done by top management from time to time throughout the year.

These review mechanisms have been very useful. They seem to be essential for a vastly spread out organization like LIC.

The amount of time spent, and the interest taken by the top and senior management in the programme is crucial to its working. While the Task Force has a significant role in formulating and in implementation of the programme, the responsibility for its success must rest with the top and the senior management.

Another important lesson from LIC experience is necessary to highlight. The management has not confined itself to the HRD sub-systems identified earlier. While assessing the impact of the programme in review meetings, the management felt the need to extend its scope from time to time. For example, while reviewing the self-development aspect of W.P.-R., the management decided that counselling training would be useful for senior managers. They would be able to make these meetings more useful by following non-directive approach. A series of programmes were introduced to train senior and middle level managers in counselling techniques. A capsule programme has been developed for Task Force members to extend the scope of counselling training. In a similar manner, role analysis programme was taken in hand and completed. The review and monitoring systems evolved by LIC have been useful in constantly improving HRD interventions in the Corporation.

LIC now also believes that the effectiveness of HRD cannot be measured in terms of business performance though, over a period of time, the improvement in the human organization must have an impact on performance. Rather, the effectiveness of HRD should be measured in terms of development of individuals. How well discretion is exercised by individuals and how they use autonomy to improve their decision-making and problem-solving skills. It would be surprising if individual growth does not contribute to improvement of performance, but the achievement of business goals alone, especially in the short run, cannot be a measure of the effectiveness of the HRD programme.

REFERENCES

Balachandran, S. (1987). *Managing Change, An Indian Experience*, Business Book, Bombay.

Dayal, I. "Role Analysis Technique in Job Evaluation," *California Management Review*, 1969, XI(4).

7

EDUCATION FOR HRD PROFESSIONALS

What should be the nature of an HRD educational programme to prepare professional in this area. A discussion of the design of the programme will have to also examine the nature of the job that the HRD functionary has to perform. I shall first examine my perception of the job and then discuss what are the essential components of training that prepare him for it.

HRD is not a functional area like marketing or production. It does not consist of a product but of an idea: The idea that individuals are capable of development. It is founded on the conviction that people are important and their involvement is necessary for an organization to be effective. This conviction is translated into practice through a variety of programmes that facilitate individual development and lead to better adjustment to the environment, develop capabilities, help towards maturing and self-reliance. The success of HRD is to be measured in terms of how organizational practices achieve or facilitate, or fail to do so, the growth of people in the organization. These beliefs and practices have to be shared widely by key persons at all levels in the organization.

The goals of HRD are achieved by supervisors and managers, though HRD functionaries would have a key role in setting out what these goals are and how they may be achieved. The managers have to be helped in evolving achievable goals. Some mangers would have to be persuaded that human development is an important part of developing an effective organization. HRD functionaries will have to analyse the situation to determine how in realistic ways the managerial practices can be developed or modified to achieve the intended goal. They would have to initiate, promote, devise and follow up HRD practices within the organization. They have a key role in these respects but achievement of goals would depend upon the people who manage and direct the affairs of the organization. For the HRD functionaries five aspects become important:

1. Examining his own assumptions about people and philosophy of HRD.
2. The understanding of social organization and politics to steer through the HRD beliefs and values among managers in the organization.
3. The ability to analyse the system and identify anchor points where HRD interventions are needed, and review of managerial practices to make them consistent with HRD goals.
4. Understanding the process of social change, and what factors account for success and failure in organizations.
5. Understanding of the HRD sub-systems.

Assuming that these are the important areas of concern of the HRD manager, and relevant areas of knowledge and skills for HRD professionals, what should the training programme cover? It should provide an opportunity to examine one's own values and attitudes towards people, society and business. The individual would have to introspect. In this introspection, help of a counsellor may be needed. A programme may have to be further reinforced and strengthened, if necessary. Additional readings by authors such as Rogers, Erikson,

Klein and others, may be assigned, and a participant may be asked to write an autobiographical account. There should be an opportunity to discuss this assignment with a qualified person designated for the purpose. There may be other opportunities for participants to take up assignments that enhance awareness of their own attitudes and values. By undertaking such an exercise, the participant would be able to crystallize his own views of man, society and work.

This exercise is even more important for practising executives. Often managers are led to conclude from immediate experience the causality in behaviour or generalize from personal experience why certain situations arise or fail to do so. In the pressure of events, one is more apt to generalize about cause-and-effect relationship. A chronic absentee is seen as an indifferent employee whereas this behaviour may be a manifestation of mismatch at work. Following the norms laid down by a union may be seen as a case of disloyalty to the organization. Repeated irritations at work may generate certain assumptions about employees and their motivation. Some of these assumptions may themselves be causes of negative behaviour. Causes and effects are sometimes interposed when viewed from the range of one's immediate experience.

The second skill for an HRD functionary is that of persuasion. As mentioned earlier, the effectiveness of HRD rests with supervisors and managers who deal with employees on a day-to-day basis. The climate of interaction in a number of organizations would have to change to bring about a new basis of relationships. Managers generally would have to examine their own assumptions about people and society. This attitude would have to reflect in how they supervise and solve problems and handle mistakes in constructive ways. Promoting and initiating HRD approaches in an organization would need patience on the part of the HRD functionary, and something akin to missionary zeal. The professional's enthusiasm, constant interaction with key managerial personnel, and inducing an examination of their motives and values have made a big contribution to a successful HRD programme. Commenting upon these issues, Sarangi (1991; p. 58) writes:

"Let me sum up a few points I have said so far.

1. Success of a change agent depends upon organizations being able to identify a person who has the right kind of attributes.
2. If a change agent does not experience growth in himself or herself through the assignment, he/she can never facilitate any change process or growth process.
3. Any training input however intellectually high it may appear to be, if the trainer does not have conviction or experience about the same, he/she will never mobilize the people or the organization. It is not only necessary that their convictions have to be strong, but there should be confidence enough in the concepts and knowledge given at the time of training; and, they are practicable and can be applied. Given a chance, one should be able to prove such convictions and confidence."

Persuading others in the organization depends as much on the professional's own conviction of HRD values, as his skill. The skill can be acquired by hardwork and practice: persuasiveness comes from internalization of his beliefs. How should the ability to persuade and communicate be developed in an educational programme? Besides a conscious effort to analyze one's own convictions, two other inputs would help: (i) study of the contribution of successful professionals, and (ii) careful examination of the individual's own successful and less successful problem solving experiences. A compilation of the work of successful HRD initiators may help, together with video cassettes on the subject. They might examine and critique live situations or interview some professionals and write about them. They must draw a distinction between the skills needed in managerial positions and those in HRD. It is not a *doing* job but one of *helping* others take up the task.

The ability to analyse the system and anchor points for HRD would need a great deal of case analysis together with readings. This aspect would have to consist of carefully chosen case material to cover a variety of oganizational situations. The purpose of these cases would be to identify the factors that critically influence organizational events so that in determining the strategy for implementing HRD, these factors are handled competently. The accompanying reading material would have to provide theoretical and conceptual understanding for analysing cases. It would be necessary to develop a system perspective for looking at organizational issues. Some of the assignments may well be live analysis of cases. A great deal of such material is becoming available. Case histories by Silvera (1988) and HRD Network compilations (1989) are useful for learning about the experiences of other organizations.

The understanding of HRD sub-systems would require a comparative study of practices in organizations. The HRD specialists would have to understand what practices have been effective and conditions under which they are successful, and how they integrate with the total system. Some field visits and write-ups of these visits would be useful. Study groups, wherever they can be arranged, could also be useful.

An HRD programme does not consist of a standard

package. Each company has to analyze its own circumstances, its history and the priorities, and develop a suitable plan of action. Most organizations have found that an experimental approach to developing a programme provides an important learning opportunity to HRD professionals. This approach is also useful for the management to choose the nature of intervention most suitable for its own circumstances. The choice of the most appropriate entry point for HRD intervention has to be considered from many angles. The management may have certain priorities; the employees or their unions may also have apprehensions about certain practices. HRD professional must encourage a careful appraisal of the sentiments associated with various aspects of the programme. It is necessary to evaluate the criticality of certain interventions for the management and the employees. Most organizations have found that testing ideas in a small part of the organization under rigorous experimental design is often useful. It gives confidence to people concerned in trying out new ideas, and builds faith in the programme.

Experimental approach allows a programme to evolve. It enables the experimenter to gain a deeper understanding of the various elements of the programme and, in many cases, enables employees to accept the programme with greater awareness of its meaning.

LIC benefited greatly by implementing their initial programme in one of the six zonal offices and covered only a small population in these offices. Assumptions were tested, as also the implementation strategy. The experience helped in bringing about many improvements in the programme.

In large organizations the programmes for educating HRD functionaries can be developed from within, with some support from external agencies. In small organizations considerable support from external programmes may be necessary. Such programmes are now available and the management will have to evaluate which of these are useful for their purpose.

Because the education of an HRD professional consists of more than knowledge and skills, he may have to involve himself personally in the total exercise of preparing himself for the job. He is not a student in a classroom in the ordinary sense, but someone who has a mission to perform. The intensity of his feeling about the mission will depend upon himself, and vary from one person to another.

The experience of Training HRD Task Force at Life Insurance Corporation may offer a useful example of training HRD professionals from within. The Task Force was created at the central office in Bombay and in each of the six zonal offices spread throughout the country. It involved around 40 officers. The main components of preparing members of the Task Force are indicated below:

1. A bibliography of books and articles was compiled and made available to Task Force members. Some of these readings were discussed in staff meetings of the Task Force in their respective offices.
2. An Initiation Workshop for five days was held for the members to include concepts, practices and experiences of HRD. The programme included assignments, role play, case analysis and skills development sessions.
3. The members worked in pairs. Invariably one member had longer experience in the Task Force who provided continuity and helped the new member adjust to the demands of the new job. They conducted two-day seminars for all officers of the divisional offices and the Branch Managers. These seminars were followed up by small group and individual meetings with officers.

4. Several of the Task Force members were sent to the Personal Growth Laboratory Programmes.
5. A second Task Force Workshop for three days was held six months after the Initiation Workshop. The concentration was on skills development, sharing of experience and discussing the research data and using it for developing action plans, including recommendations to the top management.

Several assignments were given to Task Force Members during the workshop to explore individually and in groups, the values, the attitudes and sentiments embodied in the HRD initiatives. The members had opportunity to discuss these at individual level with instructors.

REFERENCES

Maheshwari, B.L. and Sinha, D.P. (Ed) (1991). *Management of Change through Human Resource Development*, Tata McGraw-Hill, New Delhi.

National HRD Network (1989). *Towards Organizational Effectiveness Through HRD.*

Rao, T.N., Verma, K.K., Khandelwal, A.K. and Abraham, E. (1988). *Alternate Approaches and Strategies of Human Resource Development*, Rawat, Jaipur.

Sarangi, P.K. "Experience of Change Agent", *MDI Management Journal*, 1991, 5(1): 53-60.

Silvera, D.M. (1988). *Human Resource Development, The Indian Experience*, New India Publications, New Delhi.

INDEX